RADIOLOGY FOR MRCP

101 cases with discussion

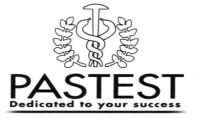

PASTEST
Dedicated to your success

This book is dedicated to our parents.

RADIOLOGY FOR MRCP

101 cases with discussion

Sarah J Howling
MB BS MRCP FRCR
Senior Registrar in Radiology,
The Middlesex Hospital,
UCL Hospitals Trust, London

Paul J Jenkins
MA BChir MRCP
Lecturer in Endocrinology,
Honorary Senior Registrar,
St Bartholomew's Hospital,
The Royal Hospitals Trust, London

First published 1998
Reprinted 1999

ISBN: 0 906896 83 5

A catalogue record for this book is available from the British Library.

The information contained within this book was obtained by the authors from reliable sources. However, while every effort has been made to ensure its accuracy, no responsibility for loss, damage or injury occasioned to any person acting or refraining from action as a result of information contained herein can be accepted by the publishers or authors.

PasTest Revision Books and Intensive Courses

PasTest has been established in the field of postgraduate medical education since 1972, providing revision books and intensive study courses for doctors preparing for their professional examinations.

Books and courses are available for the following specialties: **MRCP Part 1 and Part 2 (General Medicine and Paediatrics), MRCOG, DRCOG, MRCGP, DCH, FRCA, MRCS, PLAB.**

For further details contact:

PasTest, Freepost, Knutsford, Cheshire WA16 7BR
Tel: 01565 752000   Fax: 01565 650264

Text prepared by Breeze Ltd., Manchester.
Printed by Hobbs The Printers, Totton, Hampshire.

CONTENTS

v

COURSES INFORMATION

PasTest is dedicated to helping doctors pass their professional examinations. We have over 25 years of specialist experience in medical education and over 4000 doctors attend our revision courses each year.

Experienced lecturers:
Many of our lecturers are also examiners who teach in a lively and interesting way to ensure you:
- are familiar with current trends in exams
- receive essential advice on exam technique
- are taught how to avoid the common pitfalls
- have plenty of mock exam practice

Outstanding accelerated learning:
Our up-to-date comprehensive course material includes hundreds of sample questions similar to those you will experience in the exam. You will also receive detailed explanations, including charts and diagrams.

Choice of Courses:
PasTest has developed a wide range of high quality courses in various cities around the UK

Don't take our word for it - here's what candidates say about our courses:

'It helped me to streamline my revision studies. Thank you very much!'
Dr Lahoti, Sheffield

'Absolutely brilliant – I would not have passed without it!! Thank you!'
Dr Rajapakse, London

'Thorough, extremely well prepared – I highly recommend it. Excellent'
Dr Gordon, Southampton

'Very methodically conducted revision and exam oriented course. I strongly recommend this for any exam goer.' **Dr Ramanujachar, Swansea**

'I felt the course was excellent value for money and I would (and do) recommend it to anyone' **Dr Shawcross, Surrey**

For further details, ring PasTest on
Freephone 0800 980 9814

FOREWORD

In spite of all the changes to medical education, both undergraduate and postgraduate, over the past few years, and the massive changes in training programmes, the student and junior doctor have one constant to look forward to in their professional life: the MRCP examination. While detailed discussions have ranged over types of training, the MRCP has still emerged unscathed as the premier international examination to confirm the holder as being a competent clinician in internal medicine. The examination remains difficult but fair, and the possessor of the MRCP is acknowledged world-wide as exhibiting the best in British clinical practice.

In the past, good clinical training over a number of years was all that appeared to be required to pass the written and clinical examination, together with reasonable attention to the relevant textbooks. However, with the vast expansion of clinical medicine, particularly in its scientific aspects, the amount of knowledge required of the examinee appears to have greatly increased. At the same time, the ability to undergo training in all the relevant disciplines has become relatively difficult. There has therefore been an increasing need for text which specifically trained the examinee in many aspects of clinical medicine with which he or she may not otherwise come into contact. What has been surprising is that radiology, which has formed an increasingly important part of our clinical practise, has not had the same degree of education and attention. It is therefore a particularly opportune moment for Howling and Jenkins to have published "Radiology for MRCP", which incorporates a superb collection of radiological plates and discussion points for the aspiring candidate. Being a collaborative effort between a radiologist and an experienced clinician these cases offer excellent detailed help, and are written with great authority. Indeed, many senior clinicians may find that working through these cases would pass a highly enjoyable evening! I am therefore very pleased to be able to recommend this book, and I am sure that it will be of great value to the new generation of MRCP candidates. I wish them all the best of luck!

ASHLEY GROSSMAN FRCP
PROFESSOR OF NEUROENDOCRINOLOGY
CONSULTANT PHYSICIAN
ST BARTHOLOMEW'S HOSPITAL
LONDON

PREFACE

Candidates now preparing for the MRCP Part 2 examination need to be familiar with an ever-increasing array of imaging techniques. Although 'conventional' imaging remains the mainstay of most diagnostic imaging, there has been an increase in the use of computed tomography (CT) and magnetic resonance imaging (MRI) and this has been reflected in the types and proportions of cases encountered in the written exam.

When teaching MRCP candidates, it has become clear that access to the fundamentals of these newer imaging modalities is limited, without reference to hefty radiological texts. The 101 cases in this book, together with many supplementary radiographs, use all the relevant imaging modalities and encompass the majority of examination questions that the candidate is likely to face in both the slide section and grey cases. In most cases there is a specific answer, but in some a differential diagnosis is required. All questions are followed by a discussion and details of similar conditions that the candidate should be familiar with. This additional information may be ignored as the exam approaches, as all answers are readily identified by bold type.

Success in the examination depends on exposure to a large number of cases, which both familiarizes the candidate with the radiology of more common diseases and also encourages a stratagem for approaching those cases that are not immediately familiar. Such a stratagem is essential if all the abnormalities are to be identified on each film. It is certainly easier to see an abnormality if one is looking for it, e.g. the finding of multiple pulmonary nodules should prompt a search for rib destruction, mastectomy and mediastinal lymphadenopathy which might not otherwise be immediately apparent.

It is recommended that the candidate first reads the section on the interpretation of images at the front of this book, which is devoted to helping the reader understand the principles of interpretation, both of plain films and other imaging modalities. When appropriate, the candidate is referred to more detailed radiological texts for additional information.

ACKNOWLEDGEMENTS

The authors would like to thank Dr Katherine Miszkiel of the National Hospital for Nervous Diseases and Neurosurgery, Queens Square, London, Dr Chris Hare of the Middlesex Hospital, London and Dr Hugh Sansom of the Chelsea and Westminster Hospital, London who so willingly provided some of the radiographs reproduced here. We also thank the Department of Medical Photography at St Bartholomew's Hospital, London which prepared the photographic prints.

Sarah Howling
Paul Jenkins

GUIDANCE ON HOW TO INTERPRET THE DIFFERENT TYPES OF IMAGING MODALITIES

There is no single fixed method by which to evaluate the different types of imaging currently available. What matters is to follow a routine. What follows is the authors' own suggested scheme, with a few helpful tips on reviewing the central imaging modalities. The candidate can modify these sequences for himself.

THE CHEST RADIOGRAPH (Fig. i)

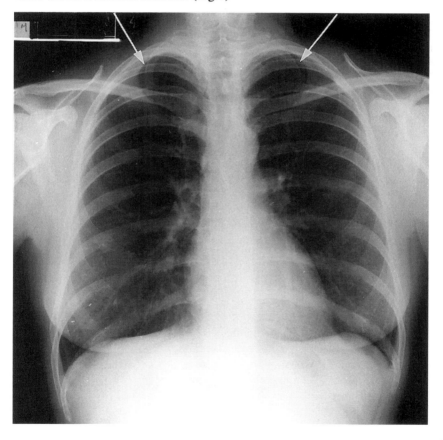

Fig. i: Normal chest radiograph. Note incidental bilateral cervical ribs (arrows).

This remains one of the most difficult plain films to interpret and an ordered approach is essential.

1. **Technical factors:** if the film is well centred, the medial ends of the clavicles are equidistant from the vertebral spinous processes. Observe the side marker and if dextrocardia is present look closely for possible bronchiectasis.

2. **Trachea:** if the trachea is not central it may be deviated away from a superior mediastinal mass (in most cases a retrosternal goitre) or pulled over to the side of the lesion by fibrosis or a decreased lung volume. The normal carinal angle (60–75°) may be widened by an enlarged left atrium or enlarged subcarinal lymph nodes. On the right the tracheal margin can be traced down to the right main bronchus. This border is known as the right paratracheal stripe (normally no greater than 5 mm wide). Widening may be due to mediastinal tumours, pleural effusions, lymphadenopathy or mediastinitis.

3. **Heart and mediastinum:** the position of the heart is variable. On average, one third lies to the right of the midline. The usual cardiothoracic ratio, i.e. the ratio of the transverse cardiac diameter to the internal, transverse thoracic diameter is less than 1:2. An increase in the transverse cardiac diameter of 1.5 cm between successive radiographs is significant. Note that apparent cardiac enlargement occurs on expiration, in the supine and AP projections and when the diaphragms are elevated. All borders of the heart and mediastinum should be clearly defined, except where the heart sits on the left hemidiaphragm. A search should be made for fluid levels, abnormal densities, mediastinal emphysema and calcifications.

4. **Hilar regions:** they should be of equal density and size with concave lateral borders. Normally the left hilum is 0.5–2 cm higher than the right. Only the pulmonary arteries and upper lobe veins contribute significantly to the hilar shadows on a chest radiograph.

5. **Lungs:** the only structures that can be visualized within normal lungs are the blood vessels, interlobar fissures and the walls of certain larger bronchi seen end on. By comparing one lung with the other, zone by zone, areas of abnormality are easier to detect. A useful rule on the lateral view is that there should be an increase in relative transradiancy as the eye travels down the thoracic vertebral bodies.

6. **Fissures:** on the PA view, only the horizontal fissure is seen. It runs from the right hilum to the region of the sixth rib in the axillary line.

7. **Diaphragm:** in most patients the right hemidiaphragm is higher than the left. On full inspiration the normal right hemidiaphragm is at the level of the sixth rib anteriorly. Loss of outline indicates that adjacent tissue has become non-air containing, e.g. lower lobe consolidation. Only the superior surface is seen unless a pneumoperitoneum is present.

8. **Soft tissues:** in females check that both breasts are present.
9. **Bones:** a survey should be made of all the bones. In particular check the ribs for notching or destruction.
10. **Below the diaphragm:** a search should be made for free intraperitoneal gas, abscesses, dilated bowel loops and a displaced gastric bubble. Calcified hepatic tumours, granulomas and gallstones may be seen.
11. **Hidden areas:** special attention should be paid to the lung apices and behind the heart.

Useful tips:
- The silhouette sign permits localization of a lesion on a PA film. An intrathoracic opacity, if in contact with a border of the heart, madiastinum or diaphragm will obscure that border, e.g. lesions of the right middle lobe or lingula will obscure the right and left cardiac borders, respectively. If, on the other hand, a border is retained and the abnormality is superimposed then it must be either anterior or posterior.
- A well-defined mass seen above the clavicles is always posterior.
- An air bronchogram indicates that shadowing is intrapulmonary.

THE ABDOMINAL RADIOGRAPH
1. **Gas pattern and position:** relatively large amounts of gas are usually present in the stomach and colon of a normal patient, with relatively small amounts in the small bowel which are rarely sufficient to outline the whole of a loop. Short fluid levels in the small and large bowel are a normal finding. The calibre of the colon is extremely variable. However, in inflammatory bowel disease a transverse colonic diameter of 5.5 cm is taken as the upper limit of normal. Look for any abnormal positioning of bowel loops which may (for example) indicate the presence of an abdominal mass.
2. **Gas outside the bowel lumen:** including inspection of the biliary tree, portal venous system, bowel wall and genitourinary system.
3. **Ascites:** should be looked for in addition to any abnormal opacities. Large masses arising from the pelvis may be due to an enlarged bladder or may be ovarian or uterine in origin.
4. **Abdominal viscera:** identify the lower borders of the liver and spleen, renal outlines and psoas muscles. Note the presence of any calcification and attempt to localize.
5. **Bones:** not forgetting the vertebral bodies, sacroiliac joints and femoral heads.

Useful tips:
- Visualization of the inner as well as the outer bowel wall – 'Rigler's sign', is a valuable indication of a pneumoperitoneum.
- Dilatation of the bowel occurs in mechanical obstruction, paralytic ileus, acute ischaemia and inflammatory bowel disease.
- The most common abdominal calcifications are of little clinical significance and include phleboliths, calcified lymph nodes, costal cartilages and arterial calcification.
- Substantial enlargement of the liver has to occur before it can be detected on a plain radiograph.

THE HAND X-RAY

Observe:
1. **Bone density:** whether normal, increased or decreased, and if abnormal, whether focal or diffuse.
2. **Soft tissues:** look for swellings, loss of soft tissues and calcifications.
3. **Joints:** assess the joint space and look specifically for erosions. If erosions are present note their site in relation to individual joints, distribution and whether symmetrical.
4. **Terminal tufts:** inspect for erosions.
5. **Alignment and deformities,** e.g. short metacarpals, ulnar deviation.
6. **Look specifically for chondrocalcinosis,** particularly in the region of the triangular fibrocartilage of the wrist joint.

THE SKULL X-RAY

The bones of the normal skull vault have an inner and outer table of compact bone with spongy bone (diploë) between them. The sutures remain visible even when fused and blood vessels cause impressions on the bones of the vault.
1. **Look for intracranial calcifications,** most of which are normal and of no clinical significance. The position of the calcified pineal gland (seen on approximately two-thirds of adult skull films) is the only means of identifying the midline. A deviation of more than 3 mm from the midline on the frontal view is abnormal.
2. **Review the bones** of the vault and skull base for areas of lysis or sclerosis.
3. **Examine the pituitary fossa.** Normal dimensions are: depth 8–12 mm; widest AP diameter of 11–16 mm. Enlargement or ballooning is most commonly due to tumours of the pituitary. The dorsum sella may be eroded in prolonged raised intracranial pressure.
4. **Inspect the paranasal air sinuses.**

INTRAVENOUS UROGRAM (IVU) (Fig. ii)

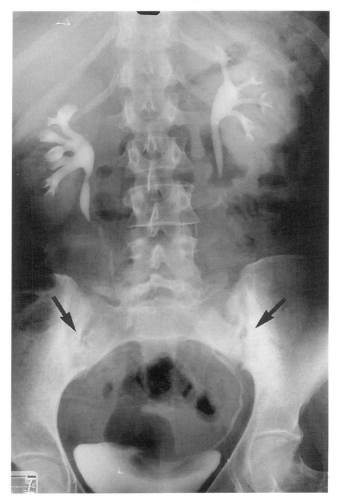

Fig. ii: Normal IVU. The smooth indentation on the bladder is due to the normal uterus. Note bilateral sacroiliitis (arrows) in this patient with a history of inflammatory bowel disease.

1. **Plain film:** identify all calcifications which will be obscured by contrast. The major causes of urinary tract calcification are: urinary calculi, nephrocalcinosis, localized calcification due to conditions such as

tuberculosis or tumours and prostatic calcification.

2. **Position of the kidneys:** the left kidney is generally higher than the right. Their axes should be parallel to the outer margins of the psoas muscles. If abnormal, the cause is most often congenital malposition or displacement by a retroperitoneal mass.

3. **Renal size:** renal length generally approximates to 3–3.5 lumbar vertebrae plus their discs. The left kidney is often slightly larger than the right but a discrepancy of more than 1.5 cm between the two sides is suspicious.

4. **Renal shape and outline:** if any indentations or bulges are present they must be explained. The renal parenchymal width should be uniform and symmetrical. A bulge of the renal outline usually indicates a mass and is generally associated with displacement and deformity of the adjacent calices. (An important normal variant causing a bulge of the left renal outline is the so-called 'splenic hump'.)

5. **The calices:** they should be reasonably symmetrical and evenly distributed. A normal calix is cup-shaped. A dilated calix is referred to as 'clubbed'. Caliceal dilatation has two basic causes: (i) obstruction – dilatation of the collecting system down to the obstructing lesion and (ii) destruction of the papilla, which may be due to chronic pyelonephritis, tuberculosis, papillary necrosis or obstructive atrophy.

6. **Renal pelves:** look for filling defects, the causes of which include calculi, blood clot, tumours and sloughed papillae.

7. **Ureters:** Only part of their length is usually seen on any one film. Dilatation is usually due to obstruction. Look also for displacement.

8. **The bladder:** shape, size and outline, which should be smooth. After micturition the bladder should be empty.

BARIUM EXAMINATIONS

1. To distinguish between a small bowel follow-through, in which serial films are taken after the ingestion of barium, and a small bowel enema, in which barium is injected through a nasojejunal tube, look for the presence of a tube which indicates that the latter has been performed. Small bowel: check the bowel calibre. A diameter of greater than 30 mm is definitely abnormal. Dilatation of small bowel usually indicates malabsorption, paralytic ileus or small bowel obstruction. Look for strictures, which must be differentiated from normal peristalsis. A smooth tapering stricture is more likely to be benign, whereas one ending abruptly, with overhanging edges giving an appearance termed 'shouldering' is more likely to be malignant. This rule is also pertinent to

large bowel studies. Inspect the mucosal folds, checking both their thickness (normally no more than 2 mm) and frequency (generally 1–6 mm apart). Small bowel folds become thickened in numerous conditions, including malabsorption, infiltration, inflammatory bowel disease and oedema of the bowel wall. Filling defects may be intraluminal, e.g. *Ascaris lumbricoides*; arise from the bowel wall, e.g. carcinoma, or extraluminal, causing wall compression, e.g. pancreatic mass.

2. Look for alteration in position of bowel loops.
3. Large bowel: note that haustra can normally be recognized in the whole of the colon but may be absent in the descending and sigmoid regions. Strictures in the large bowel are generally due to diverticular disease, Crohn's disease or ischaemic colitis and less commonly tuberculosis, radiation or lymphoma.
4. Do not forget to look outside the bowel for additional diagnostic clues, e.g. sacroiliitis, gallstones and a bamboo spine.

COMPUTED TOMOGRAPHY
Lesions of high attenuation on CT are white and have high CT values (Hounsfield Units/HU). High attenuation areas on unenhanced scans are typically due to haemorrhage (+55 to +75 HU) or calcification (+400 to +1000 HU).

Conversely, low attenuation lesions are black and have low or negative CT values. Tissues with low Hounsfield Units include air (–1000 HU), fat (–100 to –60 HU) and to a lesser degree water (0 HU).

Determining the Hounsfield Units for an undiagnosed lesion gives useful information on its composition.

- **Abdomen**

Normal appearances are demonstrated in Fig. iii. A useful approach may be to evaluate each viscus in turn, after noting whether intravenous contrast has been given (usually indicated by the abbreviation '+C') by quickly inspecting the aorta and inferior vena cava. Familiarize yourself with the normal pre- and post-contrast appearances and the density of fluid on CT (see case 85). Points to remember include:

1. **Liver:** the normal hepatic parenchyma prior to contrast enhancement has a higher density than muscle and is higher or equal in density to the spleen. The hepatic veins are seen as low density branching structures.

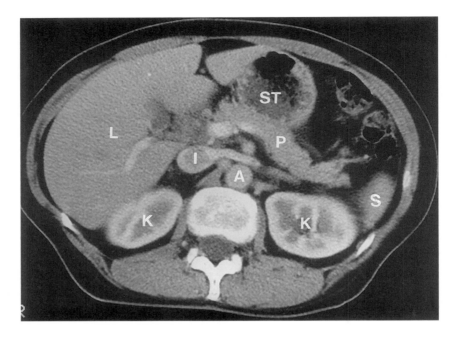

Fig. iii: Normal CT scan through the upper abdomen with intravenous contrast. Liver (L), Kidneys (K), Tip of spleen (S), Pancreas (P), Stomach (ST), Aorta (A) and Inferior Vena Cava (I).

This difference in density between the liver and spleen is accentuated by haemochromatosis and reversed by fatty infiltration. Normal intrahepatic bile ducts are not visible. Intravenous contrast is often given to emphasize the density difference between normal parenchyma and lesions which enhance poorly, e.g. most abscesses, metastases or haematomas.

2. **Spleen:** many conditions which result in enlargement of the spleen cause no change in its density on CT, e.g. portal hypertension.

3. **Renal tract:** basic principles of interpretation are the same as with the IVU. The ureters are seen as small dots in cross-section lying on the psoas muscles. CT is useful to assess renal masses, trauma, infarction and neoplastic infiltration.

4. **Adrenal glands:** the right adrenal gland lies immediately behind the inferior vena cava, whereas the left adrenal gland is normally medial to the upper pole of the left kidney. A limb thickness greater than a

diaphragmatic crus (or >10 mm) is suspicious. The adrenal glands comprise a 'body' and two 'limbs', which form an inverted 'v' or 'y' shape.

In addition to inspecting the viscera, check for ascites (fluid density surrounding the viscera), lymphadenopathy (particularly in the region of the major blood vessels), aortic aneurysm and do not forget the vertebral bodies and paraspinal regions where a psoas abscess may be lurking.

- **Brain**
1. Ascertain whether contrast has been given. It tends not to be given in patients with suspected head injury or who are suspected of recent cerebral haemorrhage.
2. Check for symmetry of the lateral ventricles and midline structures.
3. Check ventricular size. Two basic mechanisms may cause the ventricles to enlarge: (i) obstruction to the flow of cerebrospinal fluid (CSF) and (ii) secondary to atrophy of brain tissue.
4. Compare any abnormal tissue density with the normal surrounding brain. High attenuation (white) is seen with recent haemorrhage, calcification and areas of contrast enhancement. Low attenuation (black) is usually due to neoplasms or infarcts or is due to oedema which commonly surrounds tumours, infarcts, haematomas and areas of inflammation. Oedema does not enhance with intravenous contrast.
5. Do not forget to inspect the sinuses and orbits.

As a rule it is not possible to diagnose the nature of a mass based on attenuation values alone (an exception being lipoma).

MRI BASICS

- Axial, coronal and sagittal projections are all possible. Since no signal is produced from bone, there is no bone artifact and hence MRI is superior to CT in examination of the posterior fossa and spinal cord structures.
- Different sequences change the signal intensities of visualized structures. On T1-weighted images (Fig. iv), CSF appears **black** and fat appears **white**. On T2-weighted images (Fig. v), CSF appears **white**.
- High signal refers to structures that are white and, conversely, low signal structures are black.
- The natural differences in signal intensity are sufficiently great that contrast is needed much less often with MRI than with CT. If gadolinium DTPA is given then a T1-weighted sequence is performed and enhancing tissues show up as white or high signal. Enhancement implies breakdown of the blood–brain barrier.

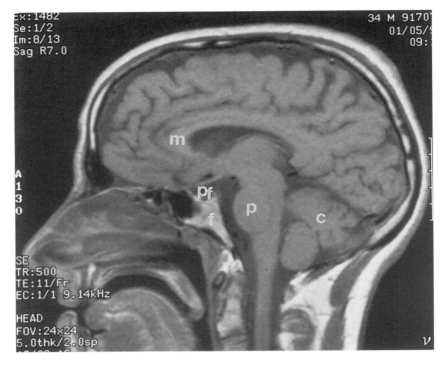

Fig. iv: Sagittal T1-weighted MRI brain scan. Cerebellum (C), Pons (P), Corpus callosum (M), Pituitary fossa (PF), Fat in marrow of clivus (F).

- MRI does not show calcification or bone detail for which CT is superior.
- Principles of diagnosis are similar to CT, in that the basic signs to look for are a change in signal intensity and evidence of mass effect.

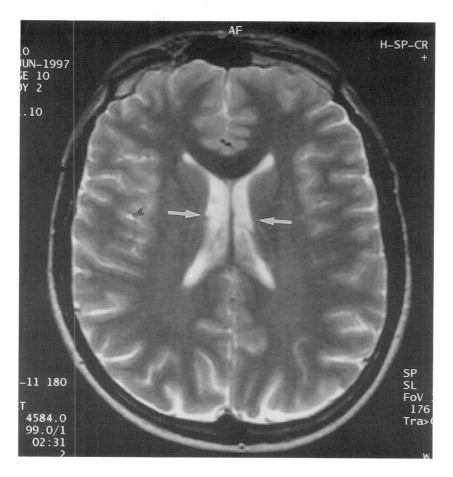

Fig. v: Axial T2-weighted MRI brain scan at the level of the bodies of the lateral ventricles (arrows).

BIBLIOGRAPHY

Diagnostic Radiology: A Textbook of Medical Imaging. Grainger RG and Allison DJ (1997) 3rd ed., Churchill Livingstone
Three volumes covering all aspects of radiology and useful as a reference text.

Clinical Imaging. An Atlas of Differential Diagnosis. Eisenberg RL (1996) 3rd ed., Lippincott–Raven
A well structured text which provides a differential radiological diagnosis for all the conditions and signs that the candidate is likely to encounter. All imaging modalities are covered and there are multiple useful illustrations.

Bone and Joint Imaging. Resnick D (1989) WB Saunders
A reference guide for all aspects of bone and joint imaging.

Aids to Radiological Differential Diagnosis. Chapman S and Nakielny R (1995) 3rd ed., WB Saunders
An excellent pocket reference book containing multiple, well explained and useful lists but no radiographic illustrations.

101 cases with discussion

CASE 1

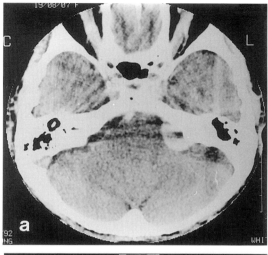

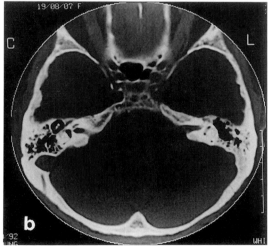

A contrast-enhanced CT head scan through the posterior fossa: (a) brain settings, (b) bone settings.

1a   Describe two radiological abnormalities.

1b   What is the most likely diagnosis in this 40-year-old patient with unilateral hearing loss?

1a   i) There is a rounded, 2 cm, densely enhancing mass in the left cerebellopontine angle. No associated calcification.

ii) Widening of the left internal auditory canal (IAC) when compared with the right side.

1b   **A left-sided acoustic neuroma**
These are typical features of an acoustic neuroma which represent 80% of all cerebellopontine angle tumours. Bilateral acoustic neuromas suggest neurofibromatosis 2. Tumours less than 1 cm in size are not consistently seen on CT, but essentially all are shown by contrast-enhanced MRI, the radiological investigation of choice. Large tumours may cause hydrocephalus.

Other causes of cerebellopontine angle masses include:
*   Meningioma (10%): hyper dense mass pre-contrast, showing dense enhancement post-intravenous contrast. Unlike acoustic neuromas they are typically larger, may be calcified and tend to be broadly based along the petrous bone.
*   Epidermoid (5%): low density mass on both pre- and post-contrast CT scans. This is the most common location for these fat containing tumours.
*   Others (5%): metastases (generally accompanied by bony erosion and a primary elsewhere), glomus jugulare tumour (associated erosion of the jugular foramen) and chordoma (most arise from the clivus).

The main differential diagnosis in this case is a meningioma and widening of the IAC is a useful discriminatory sign pointing to acoustic neuroma.

CASE 2

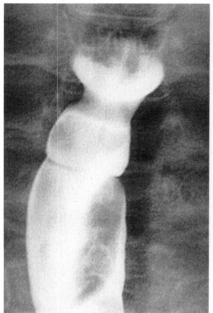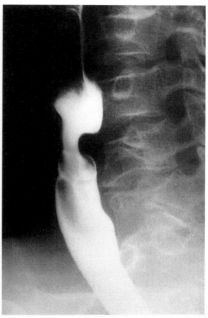

Frontal and lateral views from the barium swallow of a middle aged female with dysphagia.

2   What are the causes of the two indentations demonstrated?

2   i) **Cricopharyngeal impression:** a posterior impression on the pharynx at about the C5–C6 level, caused by the failure of the cricopharyngeus muscle to relax.

   ii) **Oesophageal web:** a smooth thin lucent band (occasionally multiple) arising from the anterior wall of the upper oesophagus just below the cricopharyngeal impression.

Oesophageal webs are semicircular membranes of variable size and are usually an incidental finding of no clinical importance, typically in the upper oesophagus. They are common in patients with dysphagia due to concomitant functional abnormalities of swallowing, but may themselves be a cause for dysphagia when large enough to produce obstruction.

Post-cricoid webs are associated with the Plummer–Vinson syndrome. The relationship to carcinoma is controversial.

Webs may occur as a complication of certain skin diseases, including epidermolysis bullosa and pemphigoid.

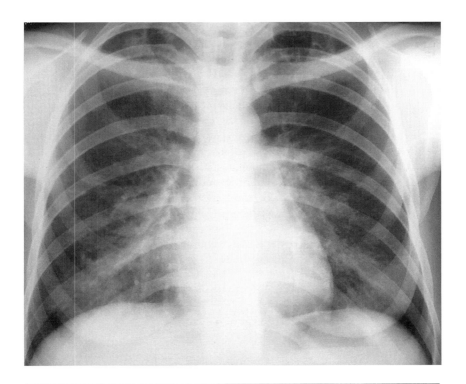

3   Give three possible causes of this radiographic appearance in a 22-year-old pyrexial patient with known malignancy, following recent chemotherapy.

3   The chest radiograph shows bilateral, perihilar air-space shadowing. The heart is of normal size and there are no pleural effusions.

The differential diagnosis includes:
- Opportunistic infection. Appearances are typical of ***Pneumocystis carinii* pneumonia** (the actual diagnosis) which is the commonest cause of opportunistic pulmonary infection in patients with the acquired immunodeficiency syndrome (AIDS). The chest radiograph is abnormal in 90% of cases, although it is often normal in the early stages. Common findings include a diffuse opacity of the lung parenchyma, which is often finely reticular in the early stages, but progresses to more confluent air-space shadowing with a tendency for perihilar accentuation. Pneumatoceles (arrow) – well defined air-spaces – may follow (Fig. 3A). Pleural effusions and lymphadenopathy are rare. Cytomegalovirus infection causes a similar appearance. Seventy-five per cent of pulmonary complications in the immunocompromized result from infection.
- Drug reaction.
- Pulmonary haemorrhage.
- Direct neoplastic involvement of the lung.

Cardiogenic oedema is unlikely given the absence of cardiomegaly and pleural effusions.

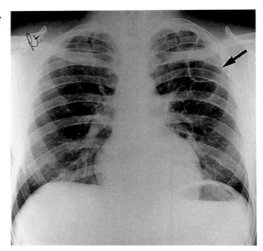

Fig. 3A. Multiple pneumatoceles in both upper zones (arrow).

CASE 4

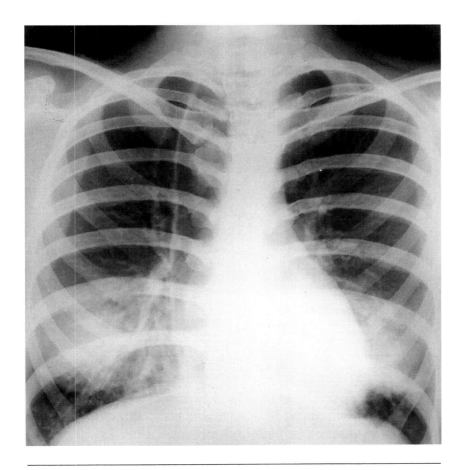

4a   Describe two abnormalities on this chest radiograph of a 40-year-old woman.

4b   What is the diagnosis and complication that has occurred?

4a i) An abnormal linear opacity extends from the diaphragm to the right of the superior mediastinum, indicating a dilated oesophagus.

ii) Bilateral basal consolidation.

4b **Achalasia** complicated by **pneumonia**, due to the aspiration of oesophageal contents.

Loss of propulsive peristaltic contractions, together with defective sphincter relaxation results in a stasis of food and a progressively dilating and tortuous oesophagus. Additional radiographic features that may be seen include an air-fluid level visible in the mediastinum (or a mottled appearance due to a mixture of air and fluid). Generally little or no air is seen in the stomach.

Barium swallow classically shows a dilated oesophagus with smooth tapering of the lower end, likened to a rat's tail (Fig. 4A).

Narrowing of the distal oesophagus is not specific to achalasia (although defective peristalsis and dilatation make this likely); it may also be seen in:
- Chagas' disease.
- Inflammatory strictures, e.g. due to reflux or corrosive ingestion.
- Neoplastic involvement: carcinoma of the oesophagus or stomach can cause an identical appearance either by direct involvement or by destruction of the myenteric plexus, although strictures are more commonly irregular.

Carcinoma is also a complication of longstanding achalasia.

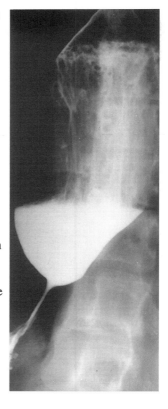

Fig. 4A. Achalasia on barium swallow.

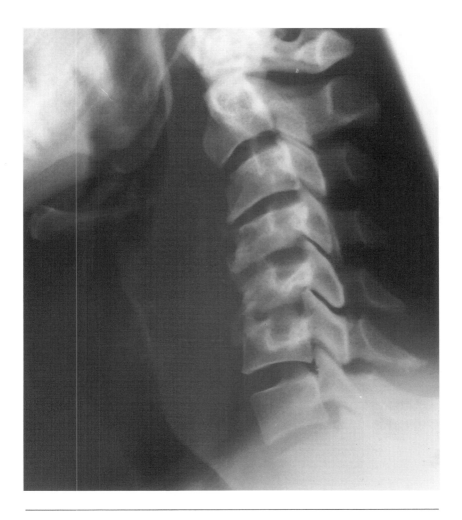

5a   What three radiological abnormalities are seen on this lateral cervical spine X-ray of an Asian man with a painful neck?

5b   What is the most likely diagnosis?

5a   i) Narrowed disc-spaces at the C4/C5 and C5/C6 levels with loss of vertebral body height and destructive foci seen in the anterior corners of C3 to C6.

      ii) Marked pre-cervical soft tissue swelling. Normally the pre-cervical soft tissues measure <4 mm down to C4, beyond which they have the maximum width of a vertebral body.

      iii)Reversal of the normal cervical lordosis.

5b   In a patient of Asian origin, appearances are most likely to be due to **tuberculous spondylitis**.

Tuberculosis typically causes irregular bone destruction in a vertebral body, with narrowing of the adjacent intervertebral disc and extension of destruction across the disc to involve the contiguous vertebral body. Unlike pyogenic infection, tuberculous osteomyelitis is often associated with a paravertebral abscess and is rarely associated with bone sclerosis, however it is usually not possible to distinguish between the two on radiological criteria alone. Calcification when present indicates tuberculosis.

The lesions generally respond rapidly to anti-tuberculous therapy and quiescence is evidenced by return of the bone detail and density and by the eroded bony margins becoming sharply defined.

CASE 6

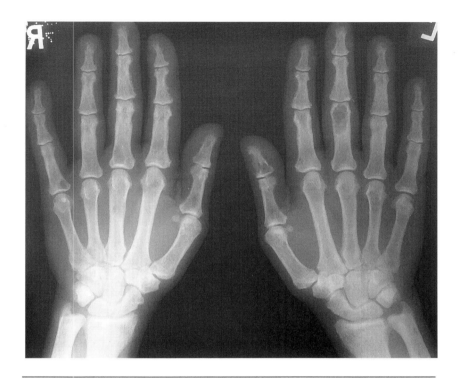

6a   What three radiological features are shown?

6b   What is the diagnosis?

6a   i) Subperiosteal bone resorption, particularly affecting the radial side of the middle phalanx of the middle fingers. Other areas that may be involved include the lateral ends of the clavicles, medial aspect of the proximal tibia, pubic symphysis and the medial aspect of the neck of the femur.

ii) Brown tumours: focal lytic lesions seen in the proximal phalanges of the left middle and right little fingers and also in the base of the terminal phalanx of the left thumb. These are locally destructive areas of intense osteoclastic activity and are most frequent in the mandible, ribs, pelvis and femora.

iii) Resorption of the terminal tufts of the phalanges.

6b   **Hyperparathyroidism**
Radiological evidence of bone disease in hyperparathyroidism is no longer commonly seen (10% of cases).

Additional radiological features that may be found include:
Bones:
• Osteopenia (uncommon).
• Diffuse cortical change – 'pepper-pot skull' (Fig. 6A).
• Bone softening – basilar invagination, wedged or cod-fish vertebra.
Soft tissues:
• Soft tissue and periarticular calcifications.
Joints:
• Marginal erosions, but no joint space narrowing. Predominantly the distal interphalangeal joints.
• Chondrocalcinosis.
Kidney:
• Nephrocalcinosis.
• Calculi (in 50%).

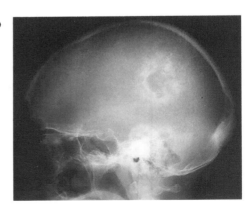

Fig. 6A. 'Pepper-pot skull'.

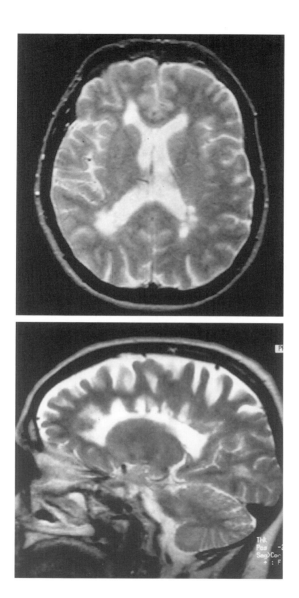

7a   What does the T_2-weighted MRI scan show in this 30-year-old female?

7b   What is the likely diagnosis?

7a   Multiple, well defined discrete foci of high signal intensity in the periventricular deep white matter of both hemispheres. The lesions are orientated perpendicular to the lateral ventricles and are not associated with mass effect.

7b   **Multiple sclerosis (MS)**
More than 85% of MS patients have ovoid periventricular lesions that are orientated perpendicularly to the long axis of the brain and lateral ventricles. The next most common site is the corpus callosum, involved in 50%–90% of patients with clinically definite MS.

In adults the brainstem and cerebellum are comparatively less common sites. Multiple lesions are typical and lesions may show enhancement with gadolinium on T_1-weighted sequences up to eight weeks following acute demyelination.

MS plaques (showing transient enhancement in the acute stage) may be seen on CT, but this is a less sensitive imaging modality than MRI.

Ischaemic lesions (areas of infarction) may have a similar appearance and patient age is useful in the distinction. In addition, the predominantly white-matter based lesions, particularly if they populate the roof of the lateral ventricles, favour the diagnosis of MS over infarction.

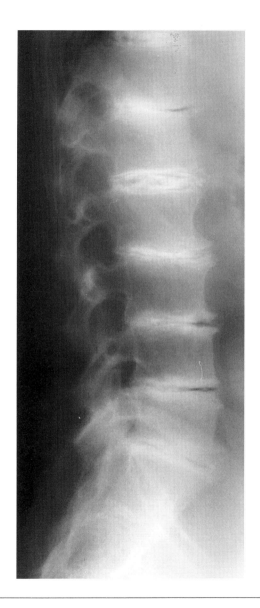

8a Describe three radiological abnormalities seen on this lumbar spine X-ray of a 48-year-old male with a stiff back.

8b What is the likely diagnosis?

8a   i) Narrrowing and dense calcification of all the lumbar discs.

       ii) Vacuum phenomenon in the T11/T12 and L1/L2 discs (air density is seen within the discs).

       iii)Marginal osteophytes and osteoporosis.

8b   **Ochronosis**
Dense laminated calcification of multiple intervertebral discs (beginning in the lumbar spine) is seen in this rare inborn error of metabolism in which deposition of a pigment derivative of homogentisic acid is deposited in connective tissues producing a distinctive form of degenerative arthritis.

Intervertebral disc spaces are narrowed and limitation of movement is common. Severe, early degenerative arthritis may develop in peripheral joints, especially the shoulders, hips and knees. Chondrocalcinosis occurs and the sacroiliac joints may be affected.

Other causes of calcification of intervertebral discs include:
- Degenerative spondylosis: a frequent finding in the elderly.
- Transient calcification in children – commonly a self-limiting finding in the cervical spine.
- Calcium pyrophosphate dihydrate deposition disease. The deposits affect the annulus fibrosus and not the nucleus pulposus as in ochronosis.
- Ankylosing spondylitis – ankylosis, square vertebral bodies and syndesmophytes also seen.
- Less commonly – juvenile chronic arthritis, haemochromatosis, diffuse idiopathic skeletal hyperostosis, gout and post-traumatic.

CASE 9

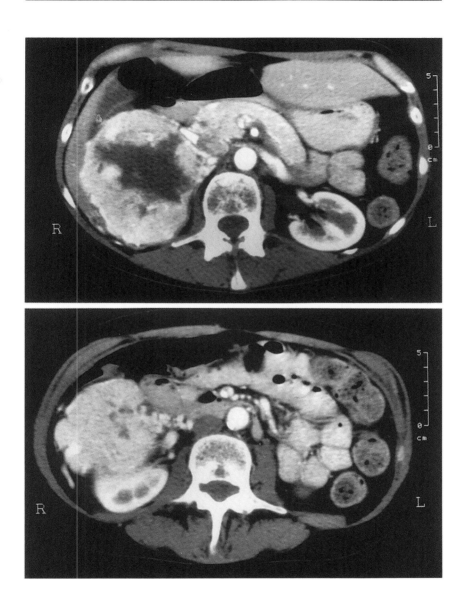

Enhanced CT scans through the abdomen in a 20-year-old girl with hypertension.

9   What is the most likely diagnosis?

9 **Phaeochromocytoma**

A large (9 cm) well defined, rounded mass is seen superior to the right kidney, which is inferiorly displaced. There is irregular rim enhancement with a central low attenuation region. The appearance is that of a right adrenal tumour with typical features of a phaeochromocytoma.

At presentation these tumours are usually large (3–5 cm) and commonly show marked contrast enhancement, either rim or patchy.

The rule of 'tens' is useful:
10% are malignant, 10% bilateral, 10% extra-adrenal and 10% are multiple. Ninety per cent are sporadic, the remainder are inherited either as an isolated disorder or as part of a systemic disease, such as multiple endocrine neoplasia (MEN IIa or IIb), von Hippel–Lindau disease, or neurofibromatosis.

Other adrenal masses include:
Benign
- 'Non-functioning adenoma' ('incidentalomas'). Occur in 5%. Generally small and homogeneous.
- Cyst. Well-defined, water density.
- Angiomyolipoma. Usually 1–2 cm and contain areas of fat density.
- Haemorrhage. Hyper-dense.
- Conn's adenoma. Generally small, homogeneous and of low density (due to cholesterol).
- Cushing's adenoma. Accounts for approximately 10% of Cushing's syndrome. Typically over 2 cm.

Malignant
- Metastases. Usually larger than 2–3 cm, irregular with patchy enhancement. Can be bilateral.
- Adrenal carcinoma. Generally larger than 6 cm, heterogenous with areas of necrosis and calcification. Can be functioning or non-functioning.
- Lymphoma. Twenty-five per cent also involve kidneys and lymphadenopathy is usually seen elsewhere.
- Neuroblastoma. Seen in infants. Calcification in 90%.

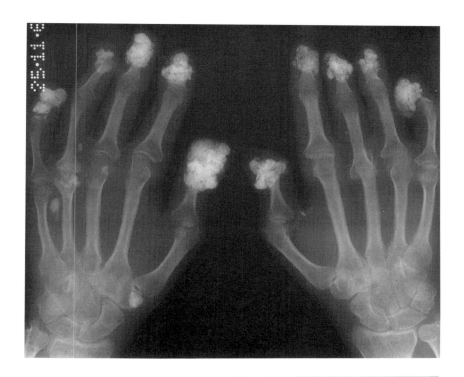

10a   Describe four radiological features.

10b   What is the diagnosis?

10a   i) Resorption of terminal phalangeal tufts.

       ii) Soft tissue calcifications, predominantly in the fingertips.

       iii)Generalized thinning of soft tissues with flexion contracture of the fingers (due to taut skin).

       iv)Reduced bone density (due to disuse).

10b   **Scleroderma**

Commoner in the hands than the feet. In 60% of cases leads to resorption of distal phalangeal tufts. Calcific deposits are associated with soft tissue atrophy. Infrequently erosions similar to rheumatoid arthritis may develop (10%).

Gastrointestinal involvement occurs in 50%, (especially atonic dilated oesophagus), interstitial fibrotic lung disease in 25% and cardiac involvement with cardiomyopathy in 35%.

Other causes of soft tissue calcification:
- Dermatomyositis – extensive calcifications may be seen in muscles and subcutaneous tissues underlying the skin lesions (Fig. 10A).
- Metabolic: hyperparathyroidism (more common in the secondary form and vascular calcification is often seen). Calcified tophi seen in gout.
- Traumatic: calcified haematoma. Myositis ossificans (outer part is more densely calcified than the centre).
- Infective: tuberculous node.
- Parasitic calcification, e.g. *Loa loa*, cysticercosis.

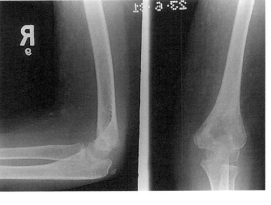

Fig. 10A. Soft tissue calcification in dermatomyositis.

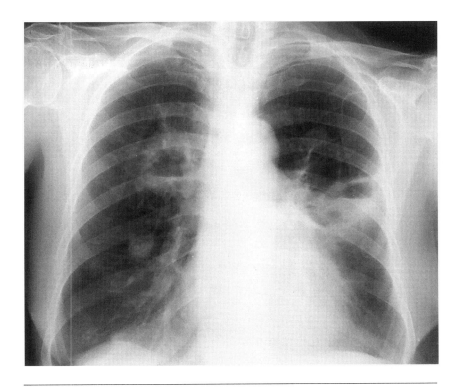

11   Give two possible diagnoses.

11   i) **Infection, e.g. staphylococcal pneumonia.**

      ii) **Wegener's granulomatosis (the actual diagnosis).**

Soft tissue density pulmonary masses, some of which are thick walled and cavitating are noted.

There are many causes of multiple cavitating lung masses:
* Infective: likely pathogens include *Staphylococcus aureus* (particularly in children), *Klebsiella pneumoniae* and tuberculosis.
* Neoplastic:
  Metastases – seen especially in squamous cell metastases (two-thirds).
  Hodgkin's disease – hilar or mediastinal lymphadenopathy generally also present.
* Vascular: Infarction – either due to septic emboli or infection of initially sterile infarcts.
* Granulomas: Wegener's granulomatosis – one or both lungs may be involved and cavitation is common (30–50%). Lesions are typically thick-walled. Nodules may be partially or completely resolved and do not calcify.
  Rheumatoid nodules – also thick-walled, especially in the lower lobes. Tend to be peripheral and well-defined.
  Sarcoidosis (rare presentation).
* Traumatic: Haematoma - usually subpleural and under point of maximal injury. Resolves slowly. Rib fractures are also often seen.

A useful mnemonic is *CAVIT*: *C*arcinoma, *A*utoimmune disease, *V*ascular, *I*nfection, *T*rauma, but ultimately clinical details are necessary to help differentiate between the numerous causes.

CASE 12

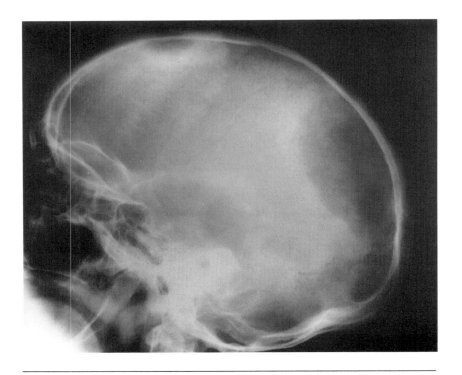

12a   Describe the radiological abnormalities shown on this skull X-ray of a 70-year-old male.

12b   What is the diagnosis?

12a   i) There is a large, sharply defined lytic lesion involving the parietal
        and occipital regions and a similar smaller lytic lesion in the
        frontal bone – osteoporosis circumscripta.

      ii) Basilar invagination. The tip of the odontoid peg is normally less
        than 0.5 cm above MacGregor's line (connecting the occiput to
        the posterior end of the hard palate).

12b **Paget's disease**

Osteoporosis circumscripta occurs in the active lytic phase of the disease and
starts in the lower parts of the frontal and occipital regions and can cross suture
lines to involve large areas of the skull vault. Later, in the sclerotic phase, the
skull vault thickens and 'cotton wool' sclerotic areas of bone are seen (Fig.
12A). The facial bones are not commonly affected. Paget's disease affects 10%
of the population in old age.

Other causes of lucencies in the skull vault of an <u>adult</u> are:
* Multiple myeloma: lesions have a 'punched out' appearance and can
affect the mandible, which metastases rarely do.
* Metastases: generally ill-defined and irregular. Common primary
tumours are breast, kidney and thyroid.
* Burr hole: well-defined. History of previous surgery.
* Hyperpara-thyroidism: 'pepper-pot' skull – which is not often severe
enough to cause
distinct lytic
lesions. Basilar
invagination may
occur and brown
tumours may be
seen.
* Infective:
(including
tuberculosis).
* Rarely:
haemangioma
and
neurofibroma.

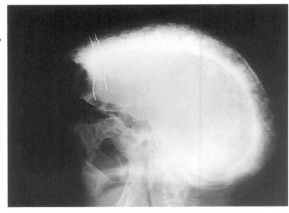

Fig. 12A. The skull is affected in 65% of cases of Paget's
disease. The hair clip is an artefact.

CASE 13

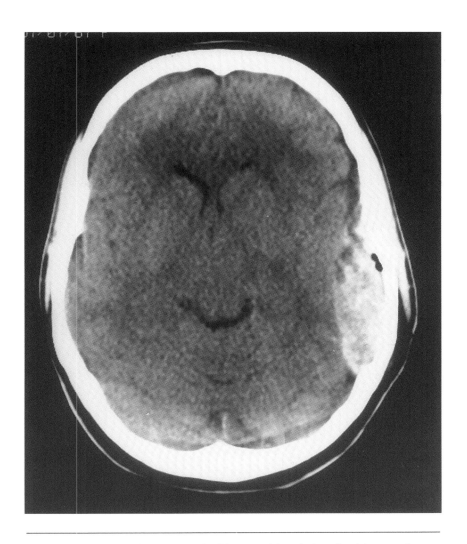

An unenhanced CT brain scan of a 30-year-old male involved in a road traffic accident.

13   List three abnormalities.

13   i) A moderate sized, high attenuation, lenticular shaped left extradural haematoma in the temporoparietal region. The heterogenous density of the collection is suggestive of active bleeding.

        ii) Intracranial air (pneumocephalus) – an air loculus is seen adjacent to the extradural haematoma. It is indicative of a base of skull fracture, or fracture through the paranasal air sinuses.

        iii)There is mass effect and shift of the midline structures from left to right.

Extradural haematoma occurs in a temporoparietal location in 66% of cases and is associated with a skull fracture in 40–85%. Note the biconvex shape compared with the crescenteric shape of a subdural haematoma. Dangerous because of focal mass effect and rapid onset.

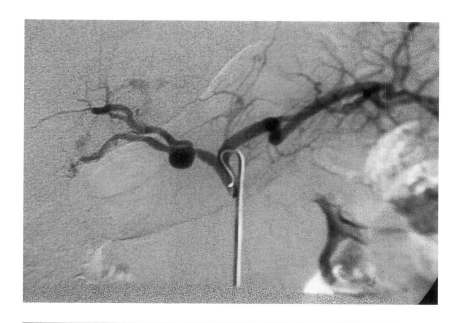

A coeliac axis angiogram of a 30-year-old female with a history of weight loss, hypertension and an elevated ESR.

14a   What abnormality is shown?

14b   Give the likely diagnosis.

14a   There is a solitary, saccular hepatic artery aneurysm arising from the common hepatic artery prior to its bifurcation.

14b   Polyarteritis nodosa

Polyarteritis nodosa is a systemic connective tissue disorder characterized by focal areas of necrotizing arteritis with aneurysm formation.

All organs may be involved: kidney (85%), heart (65%), liver (50%), pancreas, bowel, CNS (cerebrovascular accident, seizure).

Hepatic or renal angiograms show characteristic 1–5 mm saccular aneurysms, typically involving small to medium sized arteries (60–75%) and commonly multiple. The kidney may be normal in size, enlarged, shrunken from glomerulonephritis or scarred from infarction.

CASE 15

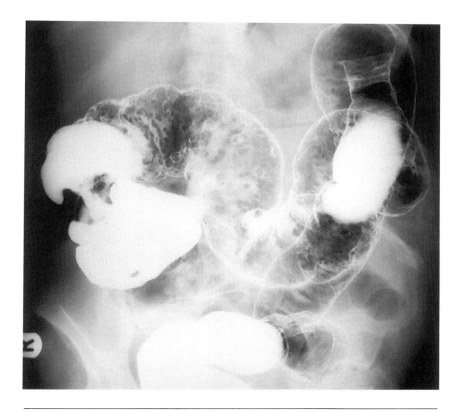

This is part of the barium enema of a 30-year-old male with abdominal pain and weight loss.

15a   What two radiological abnormalities are shown?

15b   What is the likely diagnosis?

15a   i) Multiple round filling defects are seen throughout the colon, consistent with sessile polyps of varying size.

      ii) A large annular carcinoma of the ascending colon.

15b   **A polyposis coli syndrome (familial polyposis coli) with an associated colonic carcinoma.**

Multiple intestinal polyps occur in a number of syndromes and clinical information is needed to help differentiate:
- Familial polyposis coli – autosomal dominant. Multiple adenomatous polyps (usually about 1000) appear around puberty. 2–3 mm polyps (up to 2 cm) are usually scattered evenly from rectum to caecum. Malignant transformation occurs in 100% by 20 years after diagnosis. Treatment is prophylactic total colectomy. Associated with hamartomas of stomach (49%), adenomas of duodenum (25%) and periampullary carcinoma.
- Gardner's syndrome – autosomal dominant. Characterized by colonic adenomatous polyposis (indistinguishable from familial polyposis coli). Multiple osteomata of the mandible and skull and soft tissue tumours occur. Eventual malignant transformation of polyps in 100%. Associated with periampullary carcinoma, thyroid and adrenal carcinoma.
- Peutz–Jegher's syndrome – autosomal dominant. Characterized by benign hamartomatous intestinal polyposis and mucocutaneous pigmentation. Polyps most numerous in small bowel (> 95%) compared with the colon (30%). Complications include intussusception.

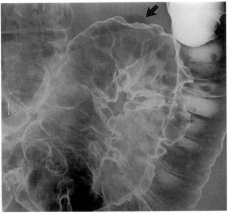

Differentiation from pneumatosis coli (Fig. 15A) is usually easy since the air cysts extend outside the mucosal line (arrow).

Fig. 15A. Pneumatosis coli. The left half of the colon is the site most commonly affected.

CASE 16

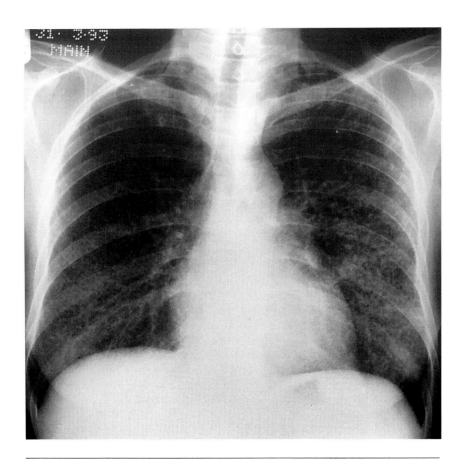

An 18-year-old patient from abroad who is unwell.

16a Describe the radiological abnormality.

16b What is the likely diagnosis?

16a   There is widespread, bilateral miliary nodular shadowing. No
        associated hilar or mediastinal lymphadenopathy.

16b   In an ill patient, **miliary tuberculosis** is the most likely diagnosis
        and the <u>pre-eminent</u> consideration as prompt diagnosis and treatment
        are vital.

Miliary tuberculosis (TB), which results from haematogenous dissemination
of the disease is an infrequent but feared complication of both primary and
reactivation TB. Radiographically, the result is widespread small (1 mm)
nodules, which are uniformly distributed and equal in size (likened in size
and appearance to millet seeds). Hilar are normal unless superimposed on
primary TB. As there is a threshold below which the nodules are invisible,
miliary TB can be present in a patient whose chest radiograph appears
normal. Even with successful treatment, the miliary nodulation may take
weeks or months to clear.

Other causes of miliary shadowing to consider are:
* Metastases: most commonly from papillary or follicular thyroid
  carcinoma.
* Coal miner's pneumoconiosis – predominantly in mid-zones.
* Fungal diseases, e.g. histoplasmosis, coccidioidomycosis.
* Sarcoidosis: predominantly mid-zones, often with enlarged hilar.
* Acute extrinsic allergic alveolitis – initially most prominent in the
  lower zones. Poorly defined.

CASE 17

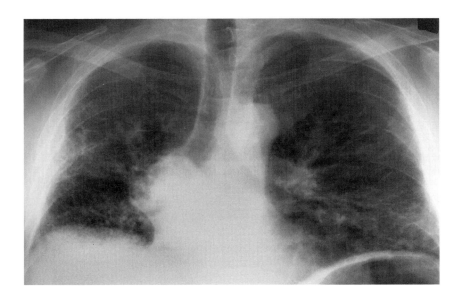

A 50-year-old male with dyspnoea and finger clubbing.

17a   Describe three radiological abnormalities.

17b   What are the likely diagnoses?

17a   i) Bilateral mid and lower zone reticular shadowing with obscuration of pulmonary vascular markings and loss of a sharp cardiac outline.

 ii) Reduced lung volumes.

 iii)Large, soft tissue density mass projected over the right hilum.

17b   **Cryptogenic fibrosing alveolitis (CFA) and bronchogenic carcinoma**

Certain radiographic features help distinguish between the many causes of pulmonary fibrosis:
*   Distribution: those conditions showing basal predominance include CFA, drug-related fibrosis, connective tissue disorders (scleroderma, rheumatoid arthritis) and asbestosis, whilst mid and upper zone predominance favours sarcoidosis, previous tuberculosis, ankylosing spondylitis, chronic extrinsic allergic alveolitis.
*   Pleural disease: calcified pleural plaques suggest previous asbestos exposure. Pleural effusions are rare in CFA, sarcoidosis and scleroderma and suggest connective tissue disorders.
*   Lymphadenopathy: 75–85% of patients with sarcoidosis have nodal enlargement at some time.

Additionally, erosion of the ends of the clavicles may be seen in rheumatoid arthritis and a dilated oesophagus (+/– air fluid level) is most suggestive of scleroderma.

In this case, in the absence of previous drug therapy, the most likely diagnosis is CFA, particularly in view of finger clubbing. Carcinoma of the lung is 14 times more common in CFA than in the general population.

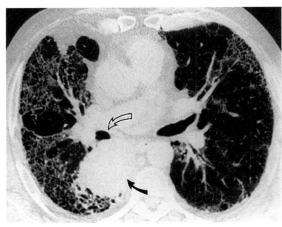

Fig. 17A. Thin section CT scan demonstrating a characteristic coarse, subpleural reticular pattern compatible with an established fibrosing alveolitis. The bronchogenic carcinoma (arrow) is seen posterior to the right main bronchus (open arrow)

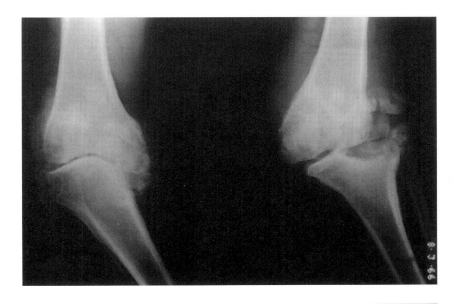

18a   Describe three radiological abnormalities shown.

18b   What is the likely diagnosis?

18c   Give a possible cause.

18a   Severe bilateral knee joint destruction, subluxation and heterotopic new bone (debris).

18b   **Neuropathic (Charcot's) joints**

18c   Tabes dorsalis.

Nothing causes as severe destruction in a joint as a Charcot's joint. The most commonly seen Charcot's joint today is in the foot of a diabetic (typically the first and second tarsometatarsal joints).

Tabes dorsalis from syphilis is now seldom seen, but predominantly affects the weight-bearing joints of the lower extremities and lower lumbar spine. The shoulder can become a Charcot's joint in syringomyelia.

Other conditions associated with neuropathic joints include alcoholism, congenital indifference to pain, leprosy, spinal cord injury and spina bifida.

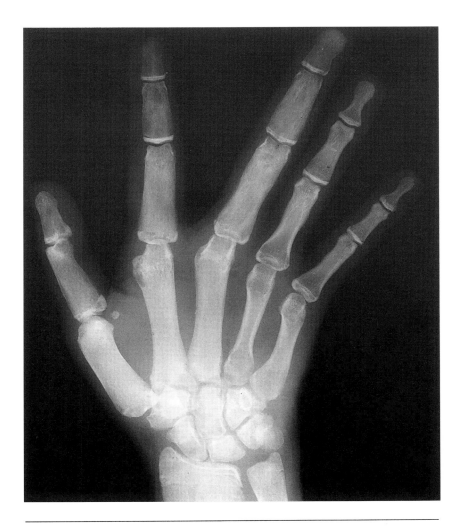

Hand X-ray of a 10-year-old girl with precocious puberty.

19a   What radiological abnormalities are shown?

19b   What is the likely diagnosis?

19a   The bone age is in advance of the patient's chronological age. There is modelling deformity of the phalanges and metacarpals with expansion of medullary cavities (especially the thumb, index and middle fingers), a thinned cortex and a 'ground-glass' appearance.

19b   The diagnosis is that of the **McCune–Albright syndrome**, with the radiological appearances being those of **polyostotic fibrous dysplasia**.

McCune–Albright syndrome (MAS) is characterized by the clinical triad of polyostotic fibrous dysplasia, café-au-lait skin pigmentation and multiple endocrinopathies. Precocious puberty is the commonest initial presentation, but other endocrinopathies that have been described include hyperthyroidism, growth hormone excess, hyperprolactinaemia, Cushing's syndrome and hypophosphataemic osteomalacia. MAS is not inherited, but occurs as a sporadic condition being caused by an activating mutation in the gene that encodes the a chain of the stimulatory G protein of adenyl cyclase, $G_{s\alpha}$.

The polyostotic fibrous dysplasia typically develops before the age of 10 years, presenting with pain, swelling, fracture or deformity. The normal bone is replaced by fibrous vascular tissue. Skull involvement may result in severe deformities, unilateral exophthalmos and cranial nerve symptoms due to foraminal obliteration.

Malignant degeneration is rare.

Paget's disease may show some similar features but affects older patients (typically over 60 years).

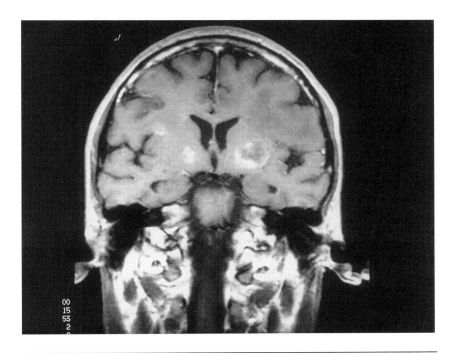

20a   Describe the radiological abnormality shown on this coronal, T$_1$-weighted, contrast-enhanced MRI brain scan, in a 26-year-old male with acquired immunodeficiency syndrome (AIDS).

20b   What is the most likely diagnosis?

20a   Multiple lesions are seen in both cerebral hemispheres which typically show ring enhancement. Lesions are seen in both basal ganglia.

20b   **Toxoplasmosis**

Toxoplasmosis is caused by the intracellular parasite *Toxoplasma gondii* and it is the most common opportunistic CNS infection in patients with AIDS. The basal ganglia and cerebral hemispheres near the cortico medullary junction are the most common sites.

Contrast-enhanced CT scans show solitary (up to 40%) or multiple ring-enhancing masses with peripheral oedema.

Lesions are typically iso- to slightly hypo-intense on T_1-weighted MRI scans. Focal nodular or rim enhancement patterns are seen following contrast administration. Treated lesions often demonstrate calcification or haemorrhage.

The major differential diagnostic consideration is primary CNS lymphoma (Fig. 20A). The detection of more than one lesion favours toxoplasmosis; periventricular location and subependymal spread favour lymphoma.

CNS lymphoma affects 6% of AIDS patients. 50% display uniform contrast enhancement and 50% show ring enhancement. Solitary lesions are present in 50% of cases and are often associated with oedema (as in Fig. 20A).

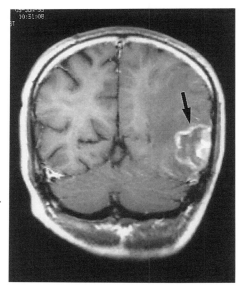

Fig. 20A. Primary CNS lymphoma (arrow) on a coronal T_1-weighted MRI brain scan.

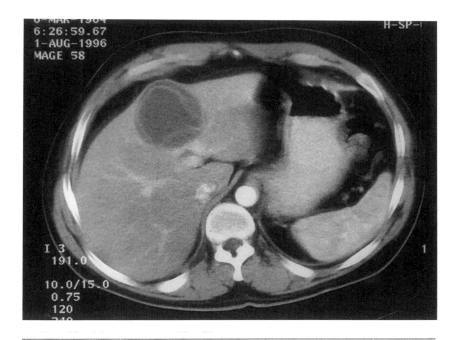

21a   Describe the abnormality seen on this contrast-enhanced CT scan
       through the upper abdomen.

21b   What is the likely diagnosis?

21a   There is a large non-calcified, low attenuation, thin-walled, cystic
       lesion within the liver. It is unilocular but a thin, wavy membrane is
       seen inside the cyst towards the periphery.

21b   **Hydatid (echinococcal) cyst**

Tissue infection of humans caused by the larval stage of a small tapeworm
for which dogs, sheep, cattle and camels are the major intermediate hosts.

A large single hepatic cyst, or multiple well-defined cystic lesions may be
seen and are often asymptomatic for many years.

On CT scan they are rounded, near-water attenuation masses with thin walls.
They may appear multi-locular with internal septations representing thin
walls of daughter cysts. Cyst walls may show dense calcification and gas
may occur within (due to superimposed infection or communication with the
biliary tree). When detached from the pericyst the true cyst wall may appear
as a thin wavy membrane (as above).

Other causes of cystic lesions within the liver are:
- Simple, congenital cyst: (common). Single or multiple. No internal
  septations. Smooth walls.
- Polycystic disease: multiple low attenuation cysts of various sizes,
  associated with polycystic kidneys.
- Abscesses: including pyogenic and amoebic. May also contain gas.
- Metastases: cystic metastases (sarcoma, melanoma, ovarian and colon carcinoma) may closely simulate benign cysts, though they often have shaggy and irregular walls (Fig. 21A).

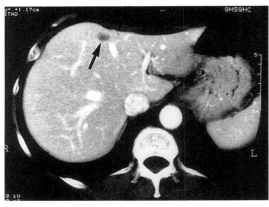

Fig. 21A. CT scan of the liver. Solitary, irregular
metastasis from colonic carcinoma (arrow). Cystic
nature confirmed on ultrasound.

CASE 22

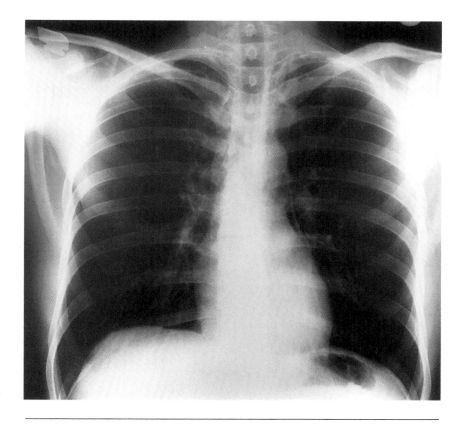

A 25-year-old presenting with chest pain following an episode of food poisoning.

22a   What abnormality is seen on this chest radiograph?

22b   What is the likely cause?

22a **Pneumomediastinum**

22b Oesophageal rupture (Boerhaave syndrome) due to excessive vomiting. Vertical streaks of air in the mediastinum are best seen in the region of the left hilum where the pleura (separated from the left hilum by air) is visualized as a linear opacity parallel to the mediastinum. The air is usually greatest in amount anteriorly and is often more obvious on the lateral view. Surgical emphysema and pneumothorax may be associated features.

The causes can be divided into:
- Alveolar rupture:
  Spontaneous – generally in healthy young patients following a bout of coughing or vomiting.
  Mechanical ventilation.
  Following compressive thoracic trauma.
  Following rupture of a lung by rib fracture.
- Traumatic laceration of the trachea or a central bronchus.
- Perforation of the oesophagus:
  Spontaneous.
  Following instrumentation.
- Perforation of pharynx, duodenum, colon or rectum with tracking of air into the mediastinum.

Symptoms include chest pain and dyspnoea. Fever and leucocytosis are frequently seen.

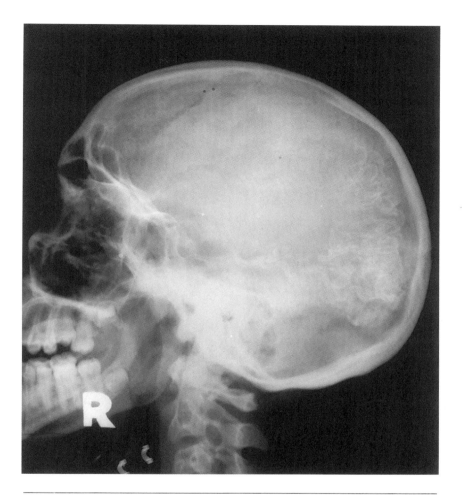

23   This young patient presented with epilepsy. What is the diagnosis?

23   **Sturge–Weber syndrome**
Characteristic tram-track, gyriform plaques of calcification in the
brain cortex that appear to follow the cerebral convolutions and most
often develop in the parieto-occipital area. They are clearly seen on
the skull X-ray.

A congenital vascular anomaly in which a localized meningeal venous
angioma occurs in conjunction with an ipsilateral facial angioma (port wine
naevus). The clinical findings include mental retardation (>50%), seizures
(90%), hemiatrophy and hemiparesis.

Additional radiological abnormalities, better demonstrated on CT scan
include: cortical hemiatrophy, ipsilateral thickening of the skull and
enlargement of ipsilateral paranasal air sinuses.

Intracranial calcifications may also be due to:
*   Physiological causes, e.g. choroid plexus/pineal calcification.
*   Infection: toxoplasmosis, rubella, cytomegalovirus, *Herpes simplex,*
    cysticercosis, tuberculosis.
*   Neoplasm: craniopharyngioma (40–80%), oligodendroglioma
    (50–70%), chordoma (25–40%), meningioma (20%).
*   Endocrine: hyperparathyroidism, hypoparathyroidism, carbon
    monoxide and lead poisoning.
*   Embryologic: tuberous sclerosis, neurofibromatosis.
*   Vascular: aneurysm, arteriovenous malformation, subdural
    haematoma.

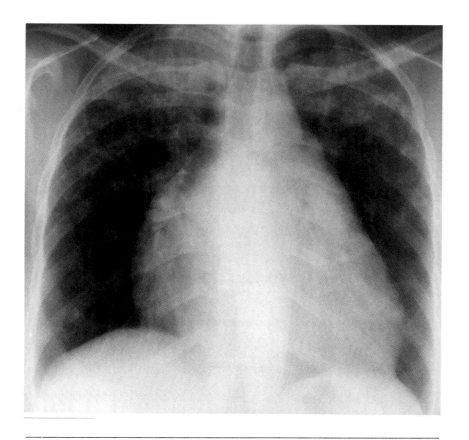

A 25-year-old male with a fever. A chest X-ray taken one week previously was normal.

24a   What two radiological abnormalities are shown?

24b   What is the most likely unifying diagnosis?

24a   i) Cardiomegaly.

ii) Bilateral upper zone air-space shadowing.

24b   **Pulmonary tuberculosis and pericardial effusion**
The rapid increase in cardiac size is highly suggestive of pericardial effusion as the cause of cardiac enlargement.

Other causes of gross cardiomegaly are:
- Multiple valvular disease – aortic and mitral valve disease, particularly with regurgitation.
- Cardiomyopathy (including ischaemic).
- Atrial septal defect.

Plain film appearances depend on the amount of pericardial fluid present. The cardiac silhouette may be globular or have a non-specific shape, but with no specific features to suggest selective chamber enlargement (as will be the case in some of the other causes listed). Abnormalities of pulmonary vasculature are striking by their absence.

Causes of a pericardial effusion include:
- Infective (bacterial, tuberculous or viral)
- Malignancy
- Dressler's syndrome
- Myxoedema
- Systemic lupus erythematosus
- Uraemia
- Trauma.

Consolidation in the upper zones in an Asian patient with a fever should suggest the possibility of tuberculosis.

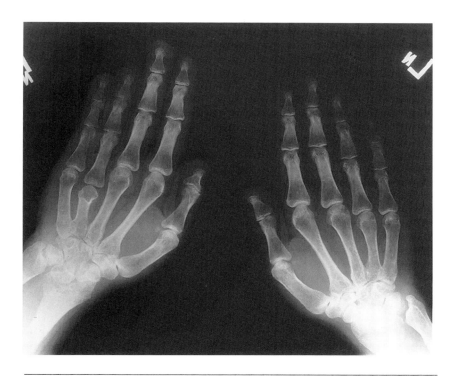

25   List three possible causes of this appearance.

25   i) **Pseudohypoparathyroidism**

ii) **Pseudopseudohypoparathyroidism**

iii)**Turner's syndrome**

There is shortening of the right and (to a lesser extent) the left fourth metacarpals. A tangent between the third and fifth metacarpals normally intersects the fourth.

The principal radiological findings in pseudohypoparathyroidism are short stature with short metacarpals, metatarsals and phalanges, particularly the fourth and fifth metacarpals. Calcification may be present in the basal ganglia, cerebellum and skin.

Pseudopseudohypoparathyroidism presents the same skeletal syndrome, but with normal blood chemistry.

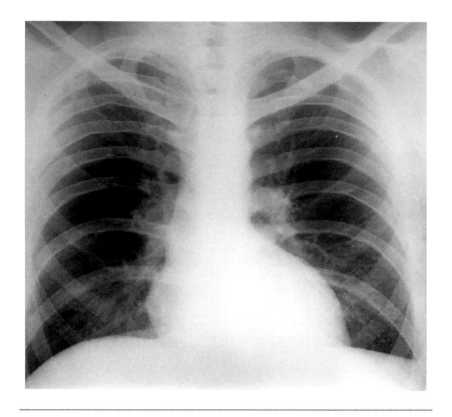

A 26-year-old male found to be hypertensive at an insurance medical examination.

26a   What is the likely diagnosis?

26b   Name three associations.

26a **Coarctation of the aorta**
There is notching of the inferior aspects of the posterior ribs
bilaterally, sparing the upper two ribs. The heart is not enlarged but
the aortic knuckle has an abnormal 'figure 3' configuration.

26b i) Turner's syndrome (13–15% of female patients).

ii) Bicuspid aortic valve (50%).

iii)Cerebral berry aneurysms.

Coarctation of the aorta refers to an area of localized narrowing. It is most
commonly congenital and may be either pre-ductal or post-ductal in
location.

The chest radiograph shows rib notching (caused by dilatation and tortuosity
of the intercostal arteries) affecting the inferior surfaces of the posterior rib
elements, but not usually seen before the second decade. Generally rib
notching is bilateral and spares the first two ribs.

The aortic knuckle can have an abnormal 'figure 3' configuration caused by
the dilated origin of the left subclavian artery and post-stenotic dilatation of
the arch.

Cardiomegaly suggests associated aortic valve disease and signs of cardiac
failure may be present.

Other causes of inferior rib notching include:
• Neurofibromatosis – 'ribbon ribs' may also be a feature.
• Superior vena cava obstruction.
• Pulmonary oligaemia – any cause of decreased pulmonary blood
  supply.
• Subclavian obstruction – most commonly post-Blalock operation for
  Fallot's tetralogy, which typically leads to unilateral rib notching of
  the upper three or four ribs on the operation side.

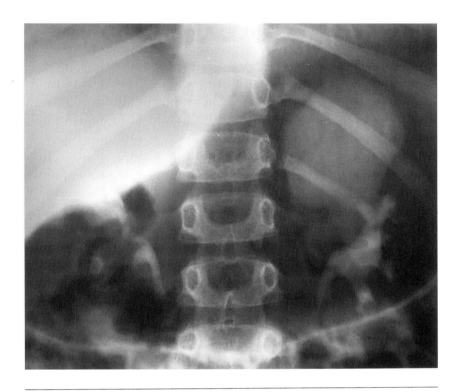

27   Describe two abnormalities shown on this IVU of a child.

27   i) Large left kidney.

     ii) **Duplication of the left renal pelvis and ureter (duplex) with hydronephrosis of the upper pole moiety.**

Complete duplication occurs in 0.5–10% of live births and in 15–40% of cases is bilateral. The ureter from the upper pole moiety inserts below and medial to the ureter from the lower pole moiety and is subject to obstruction. A ureterocele is commonly associated. In the presence of a hydronephrotic upper moiety, lower moiety calyces may have a 'drooping flower' appearance.

In some cases, the ureter may drain into the vagina or bladder neck.

The lower pole moiety is subject to vesicoureteral reflux and may atrophy secondary to chronic pyelonephritis.

CASE 28

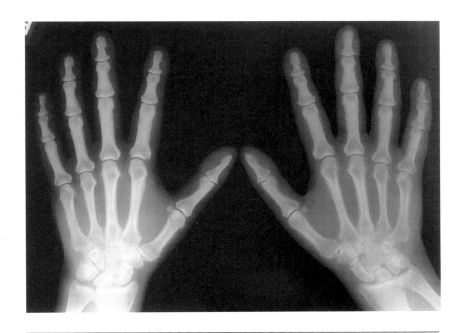

A 50-year-old female with a history of thyroidectomy 10 years previously and now presenting with painless, swollen hands.

28a What abnormality is shown?

28b What is the diagnosis?

28a   Vertical, spiculated and feathery dense bone is seen along the shafts
       of the proximal phalanges due to periosteal reaction.

28b   **Thyroid acropachy**

Thyroid acropachy occurs in 0.5–10% of patients following thyroidectomy
for hyperthyroidism and who may be euthyroid, hypothyroid or
hyperthyroid. It mainly affects the proximal phalanges in the hands; less
commonly the feet, lower legs and forearms are involved. The extremities
may be swollen or clubbed.

Causes of bilaterally symmetrical periosteal reaction in adults include:
*   Hypertrophic osteoarthropathy (HOA). Thick, irregular undulating
    periosteal reaction. It involves the shafts of tubular bones (especially
    the long bones of the forearm and leg), sparing the ends. Involvement
    of the hands is less common.
*   Pachydermoperiostitis – a rare, self-limiting and familial condition
    that most commonly affects adolescent males. Compared with HOA
    it is relatively pain free. Periosteal reaction also affects the bone ends
    but otherwise has the same favoured distribution as HOA.
*   Vascular insufficiency – the legs are affected almost exclusively.
    Phleboliths may be seen.
*   Fluorosis – solid, undulating periosteal reaction. However, the bones
    are dense and ligamentous calcification is often present.

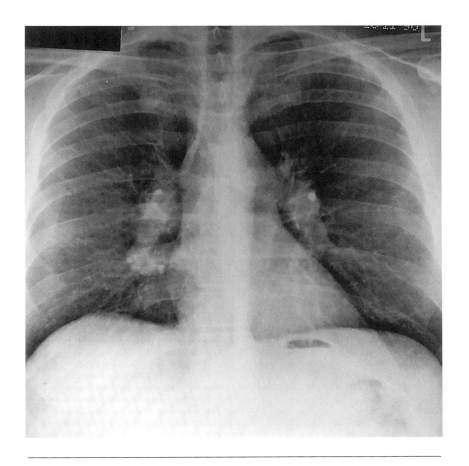

29a   Describe two radiological abnormalities on this chest X-ray of a 35-year-old male with a chronic cough.

29b   What is the most likely diagnosis?

29a   i) Bilateral, symmetrical hilar lymphadenopathy with some associated calcification.

       ii) A fine nodular infiltrate in both lungs, predominantly in the mid-zones.

29b   **Sarcoidosis**

At clinical presentation the chest radiograph in patients with sarcoidosis may be:
- Normal 8%
- Bilateral hilar lymphadenopathy 50%
- Bilateral hilar lymphadenopathy + pulmonary infiltrate 30%
- Pulmonary infiltrate ± fibrosis 12%.

Hilar lymphadenopathy is generally symmetrical and often accompanied by right paratracheal nodes. Rarely, hilar lymphadenopathy is unilateral (3–5%). Calcification of hilar nodes occurs in 5% of patients and can be punctate or 'egg-shell'.

Lung parenchymal shadowing predominantly occurs in the mid and upper zones.

Other causes of bilateral hilar enlargement are:
- Enlarged lymph nodes:
  Lymphoma (50% in Hodgkin's disease). Generally asymmetrical, unlike sarcoid.
  Metastases. Generally unilateral.
  Tuberculosis. Rarely bilateral and symmetrical.
  Less commonly leukaemia, silicosis and viral infections in childhood.
- Enlarged blood vessels.
- Pulmonary arterial hypertension.

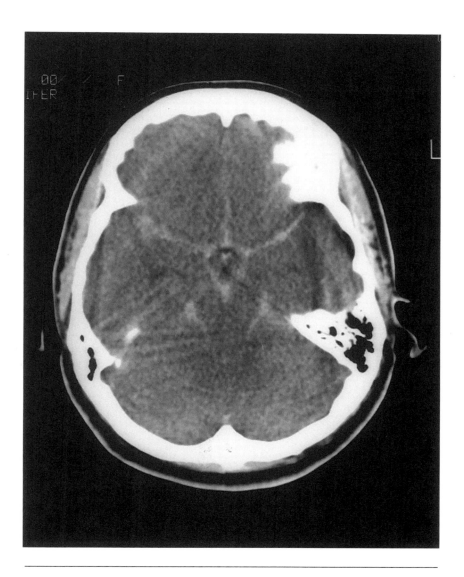

Unenhanced CT head scan of a 20-year-old with a severe headache.

30a   What is the diagnosis?

30b   What complication may occur and be visible on CT scanning?

30a **Subarachnoid haemorrhage (SAH)**
High attenuation material (blood) is seen within the basal cisterns.

30b Hydrocephalus

Non-contrast CT scanning is the imaging modality of choice to detect acute SAH with a sensitivity of 90% in the first 24 hours, declining thereafter, with persistence of blood after four days only seen in massive haemorrhage. MRI is relatively insensitive.

Increased density may be seen with the sulci (which may therefore no longer be visible), basal cisterns, sylvian fissures or ventricles and is often maximal near to the site of bleeding. If blood extends into the interhemispheric fissure this may appear abnormally thickened.

Complications include hydrocephalus, cerebral infarction (due to vasospasm) and oedema.

SAH is due to a ruptured aneurysm in 75% of cases, which can be demonstrated on cerebral angiography (Fig. 30A) or magnetic resonance angiography; 20% are multiple.

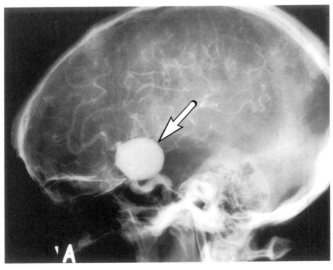

Fig. 30A. Large 'berry' aneurysm (arrow) arising from the circle of Willis.

CASE 31

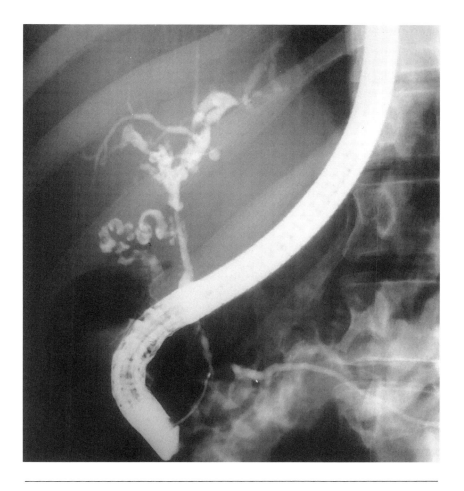

31a   What type of study is demonstrated?

31b   What is the likely diagnosis in this 38-year-old female?

31a   Endoscopic retrograde cholangio pancreatography (ERCP).

31b   Sclerosing cholangitis.
Both the common bile duct and pancreatic duct are filled with contrast. There are multiple strictures affecting the extra- and intra-hepatic ducts with slight to moderate dilatation of the intervening duct segments.

About one-third of cases of sclerosing cholangitis have coexistent inflammatory bowel disease (usually ulcerative colitis).

Complications include biliary cirrhosis, portal hypertension and cholangiocarcinoma (12%).

Other causes of multiple biliary strictures are:
- Primary biliary cirrhosis – disease limited to intra-hepatic ducts (unlike in sclerosing cholangitis which affects both intra- and extra-hepatic ducts in 90%) and strictures are less pronounced.
- Cholangiocarcinoma – usually a short, well-demarcated narrowing of the bile duct and only very rarely multi-centric.
- Recurrent pyogenic cholangitis – variable picture. History usually helpful.

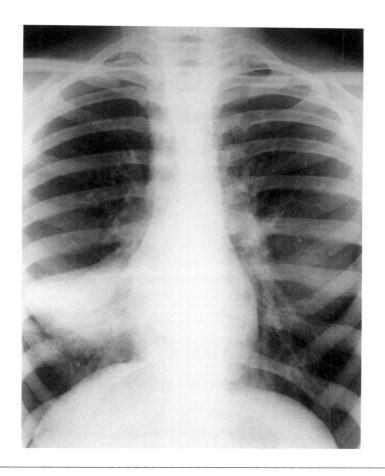

A young asthmatic patient presenting with a cough.

32   What is the cause of this abnormal chest radiograph?

32   **Collapse/consolidation of the right middle lobe**

Most probably secondary to mucous plug obstruction. The diagnosis is confirmed on the lateral film (Fig. 32A).

In middle lobe collapse, the horizontal fissure and lower half of the oblique fissure move towards one another – best seen in the lateral projection. Obscuration of the right heart border is often present, particularly when there is associated consolidation. Since the volume of the middle lobe is relatively small, indirect signs of volume loss, including elevation of the hemidiaphragm, mediastinal or hilar displacement and compensatory hyper-inflation, are rarely present.

Each lobe collapses in a characteristic fashion (Figs. 32B and 32C) and radiological clues as to the cause of the collapse may be present, e.g. enlarged lymph nodes, bronchogenic carcinoma or an inhaled foreign body.

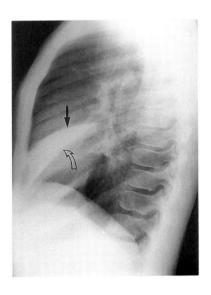

Fig. 32A. Lateral view – right middle lobe
collapse/consolidation. Horizontal fissure (arrow) and right
oblique fissure (open arrow) are approximated.

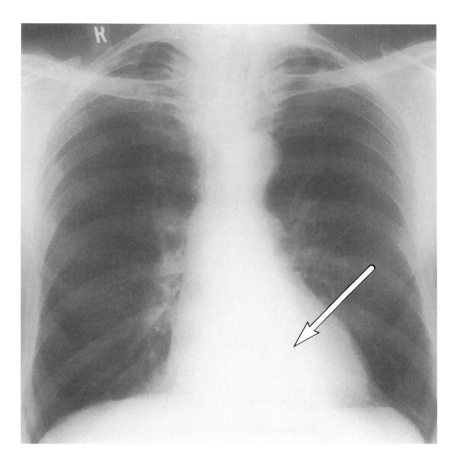

Fig. 32B. Left lower lobe collapse. Note the triangular density behind the cardiac silhouette (arrow).

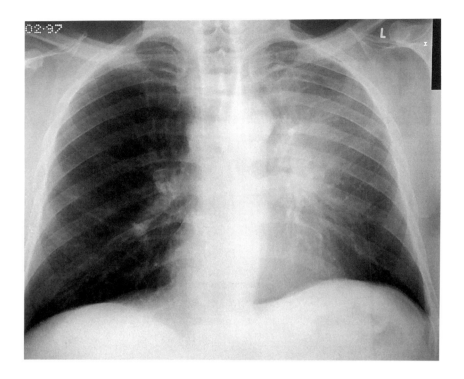

Fig. 32C. Left upper lobe collapse, with the characteristic 'veiling' effect and raised left hemidiaphragm. A left hilar carcinoma was the cause.

CASE 33

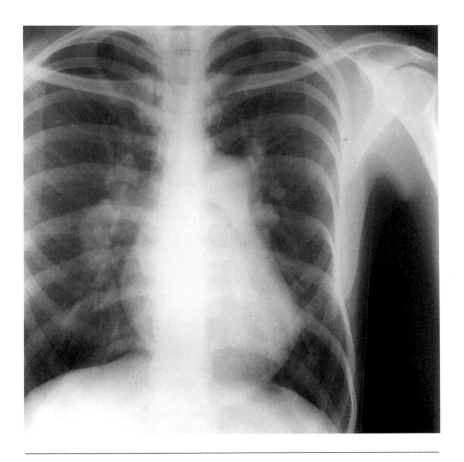

33a   Describe three radiological abnormalities.

33b   What is the most likely diagnosis in this 36-year-old cyanosed male?

33a   i) Cardiomegaly.

     ii) Dilation of the central pulmonary arteries. The peripheral vessels appear 'pruned'.

     iii)Small aortic arch.

33b   **Eisenmenger syndrome**, due to atrial septal defect.

The Eisenmenger syndrome refers to reversal of a shunt at whatever site, resulting from pulmonary arterial hypertension.

Chest radiograph appearances may provide clues as to the site of the defect.

With atrial septal defects (ASD) the heart size is often very enlarged with a small aortic knuckle (due to cardiac rotation) and the main pulmonary arteries may be markedly dilated.

With ventricular septal defects (VSD) the heart size is either normal or slightly enlarged and the pulmonary trunk is only minimally dilated. Distal vessel pruning occurs more gradually than ASD. The left atrium will be enlarged, but in many cases the chest radiograph appears normal.

Eisenmenger syndrome occurs in 2% of large VSDs by two years of age.

In ductus arteriosus defects, cardiac size mimics VSD, but the aortic knuckle is generally enlarged.

Causes of a small aortic arch are:
*   Decreased cardiac output, e.g. mitral stenosis.
*   ASD (left to right intracardiac shunt).
*   Coarctation – long segment 'infantile type'.

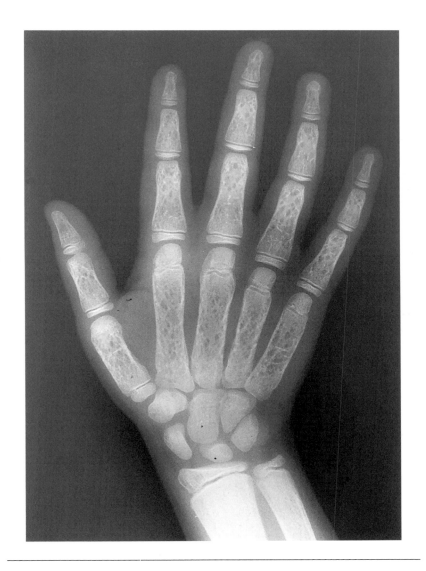

Hand X-ray of a 12-year-old boy.

34a   What is the likely diagnosis?

34b   What other radiological abnormalities may be seen in this condition?

34a **Thalassaemia major**

Marrow hyperplasia destroys many of the medullary trabeculae and expands and thins the overlying cortex. In children, this process is especially evident in the hands, when the shafts of the phalanges and metacarpals become biconvex instead of biconcave.

34b Other radiological abnormalities seen in thalassaemia major are:
* Skull – (Fig. 34A) widening of the diploic space, thinning of the outer table and a 'hair-on-end' appearance. Involvement of the facial bones produces obliteration of the paranasal sinuses, mastoid air cells, as well as lateral displacement of the orbits.
* Chest – cardiac enlargement and congestive cardiac failure. Paravertebral masses (= extramedullary haematopoiesis).
* Spine – osteoporosis, exaggerated vertical trabeculae and fish-shaped vertebrae.
* Ribs, clavicles, feet – typical changes of marrow hyperplasia.

Marrow hyperplasia in beta-thalassaemia is more pronounced than in sickle cell anaemia and with facial bone changes rarely occurring in the latter, an important differentiating sign.

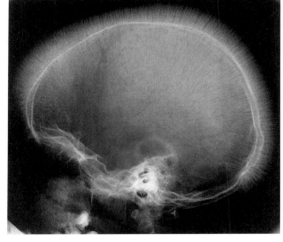

Fig. 34A. Lateral skull, 'hair-on-end' appearance. Note the normal calvarium inferior to the internal occipital protuberance (marrow content here is minimal). Poor pneumatization of the sinuses.

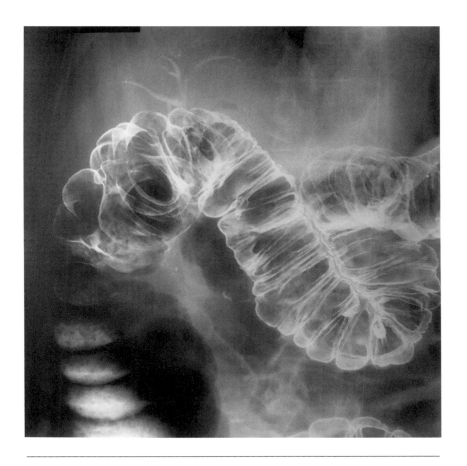

35   What abnormality is shown on this film from a barium enema series?

35   **A biliary–colic fistula**
Barium outlines both the transverse colon and biliary tree indicating the presence of a biliary–enteric fistula.

Other biliary–enteric fistulae may be encountered:
- Cholecystoduodenal fistula (50–70%) – passage of a gallstone from an inflamed gallbladder directly into the bowel may result in a fistula; associated with gallstone ileus in 20%.
- Choledochoduodenal fistula (15%).
- Multiple fistulae (15%).

Aetiologies include cholelithiasis (90%), acute/chronic cholecystitis, biliary tract carcinoma, regional invasive neoplasia, diverticulitis, inflammatory bowel disease and trauma.

Abnormal barium filling of the biliary tree may be also seen post-surgery, e.g. choledochoduodenostomy and with a patulous sphincter of Oddi on an upper gastrointestinal barium study.

CASE 36

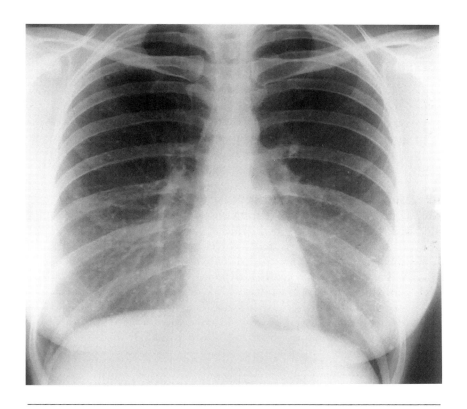

36a What abnormality is shown on the chest radiograph of an asymptomatic 42-year-old female?

36b What is the likely explanation?

36a   Multiple, well-defined, randomly scattered, small (2–3 mm), dense calcifications in otherwise normal appearing lungs.

36b   **Previous chickenpox pneumonia**

Over 90% of cases of varicella–zoster pneumonia occur in adults, particularly in those who are immunocompromized. In the acute phase (one to six days after the onset of the skin rash), the pneumonia causes multiple small ill-defined nodules, which may come and go in different areas of the lungs. In a few patients, these nodules calcify.

Other causes of diffuse pulmonary calcifications include:
- Healed histoplasmosis – in endemic areas there may also be multiple punctate calcifications in the spleen.
- Tuberculosis – nodules have a tendency to aggregate, particularly in the upper zones.
- Chronic pulmonary venous hypertension – especially mitral stenosis.
- Calcifying/ossifying metastases – including osteosarcoma, chondrosarcoma, mucinous adenocarcinoma of the colon or breast, papillary carcinoma of the thyroid and carcinoid.
- Alveolar microlithiasis (Fig. 36A) – often familial. Myriad minute calcifications in alveoli which obscure all lung detail.

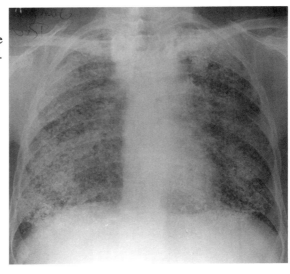

Fig. 36A. Alveolar microlithiasis.

CASE 37

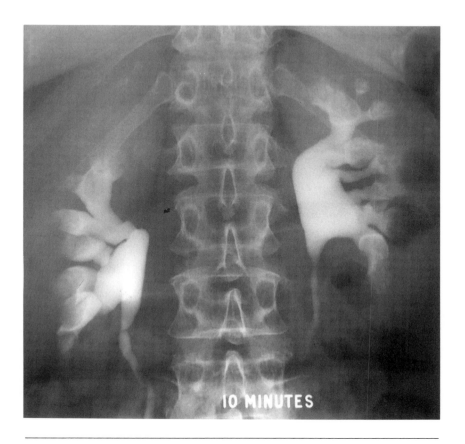

A 35-year-old female with a previous history of renal colic.

37   What is the diagnosis?

37   Medullary sponge kidneys

Medullary sponge kidney is a congenital cystic disease of the medulla resulting in localized dilatations of the collecting ducts in the papillae. Part or all of one or both kidneys may be involved and in 75% of cases the changes are bilateral.

Plain films show calcification in up to 80% of affected patients. The characteristic appearance is of clustered small opacities (1–2 mm) visualized in the region of the papillae, the 'bunch of grapes' appearance.

Most cases are diagnosed on IVU: contrast examination characteristically reveals thick, dense streaks of contrast, 'bunch of flowers', radiating peripherally from pyramids. The affected calyces are often broader than normal and, similarly, the kidneys may be enlarged.

The differential diagnosis of abnormally shaped calyces also includes:
- Normal variant – 'papillary blush' – but without distinct streaks or nephrocalcinosis.
- Renal tuberculosis – calcifications tend to be more irregular and larger and strictures are usually evident.
- Chronic pyelonephritis – clubbed, dilated calyces with cortical scarring overlying involved calyces.
- Hydronephrosis – dilatation of the entire pelvo-calyceal system.
- Papillary necrosis – no distinct streaks.
- Congenital megacalyces. Renal size is normal. Calyces often appear multi-faceted.

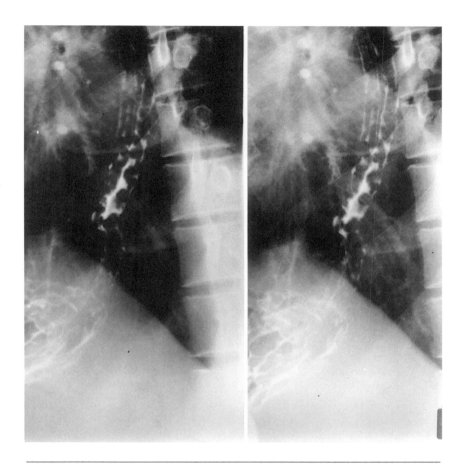

This is a barium swallow of a 32-year-old man with haematemesis.

38   What is the likely diagnosis?

38   **Oesophageal varices**
Diffuse, round and serpiginous filling defects in the distal
oesophagus, reflecting dilated submucosal veins.

The distal oesophagus is involved in portal hypertension. 'Downhill' varices
in the upper oesophagus are due to superior vena cava obstruction.

Demonstration of varices does not necessarily establish the cause of
haematemesis since one-third of such patients bleed from other causes, e.g.
peptic ulcer. Endoscopy is the preferred investigation of choice.

Other causes of filling defects in the distal oesophagus are:
- Oesophagitis – can simulate the appearance of varices. Clinical
  details are usually helpful in differentiating. In oesophagitis there is
  usually a mucosal abnormality in addition to thickened folds. When
  due to reflux there is often also a hiatus hernia present.
- Carcinoma – fixed, thickened mucosal folds seen in the varicoid
  cancer form.
- Lymphoma – rarely presents as a submucosal tumour. Generally
  evidence of lymphoma elsewhere.

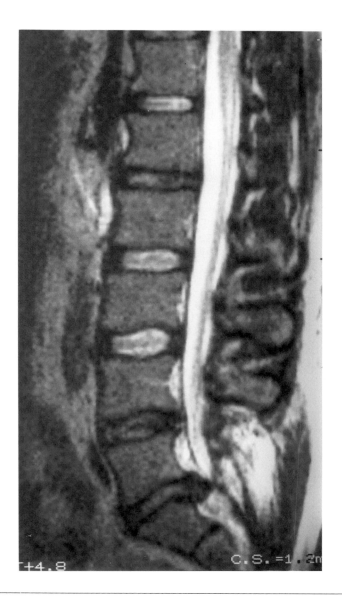

A sagittal T$_2$-weighted MRI scan of the lumbar spine.

39   What abnormality is shown?

39   **A large L5/S1 disc herniation**, of low signal intensity compressing the thecal sac. Note the abnormal low signal at the L1/L2, L4/L5 and L5/S1 levels in keeping with degenerate disc disease. Compare with the normal high signal L3/L4 disc.

Disc herniation (focal protrusion of disc material beyond the margins of the adjacent vertebral endplates through a defect in the annulus fibrosus) is common. By age 60, nearly one-third of asymptomatic patients have one or more disc herniations. Approximately 90% occur at L4/L5 or L5/S1 levels and are most commonly posterolateral protrusions.

Other signs of degenerative disc disease on MRI are narrowing of disc spaces and decreased signal on T_2-weighted scans. Disc material can detach and migrate away from the parent disc. These so-called free fragments are easily detected on MRI scans and cephalad and caudal extension occur approximately equally.

CASE 40

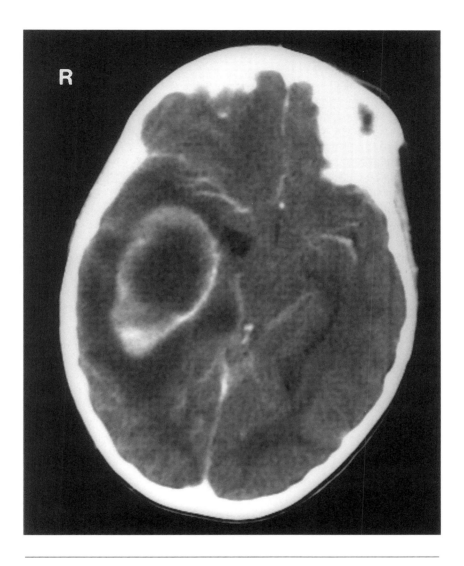

An enhanced CT head scan of a pyrexial 38-year-old patient.

40a   What abnormality is shown?

40b   What is the diagnosis?

40a   There is ring enhancement of a large mass in the right temporo-parietal region associated with cerebral oedema and mass effect.

40b   The appearances in a pyrexial patient are most likely to represent **cerebral abscess**.

The commonest causes of a cerebral abscess are trauma and direct extension from an infected sinus. In up to 30% of cases, abscesses are multiple. CT scanning shows a heterogeneous mass of low attenuation with oedema and loculi may be evident. Ninety per cent of abscesses show contrast enhancement, generally as a peripheral, thin, smooth ring. The relatively poor inflammatory response of deep hemispheric white matter may cause the capsule of an abscess to be better developed along the medial wall.

Other causes of cerebral ring-enhancing masses are:

- Metastases – irregular rim enhancement and typically located at the grey-white matter junction; multiple in 50% of cases (Fig. 40A).
- Lymphoma – single or multiple ring enhancing lesions.
- Glioblastoma multiforme. Thick irregular ring enhance-ment in a solitary lesion that tends to be situated in a deep hemispheric location. Rarely multi-centric.

Note that oedema and also contrast enhancement may be suppressed by steroids.

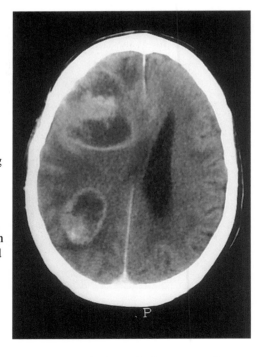

Fig. 40A. Multiple cerebral metastases from carcinoma of the breast. There is considerable associated oedema.

CASE 41

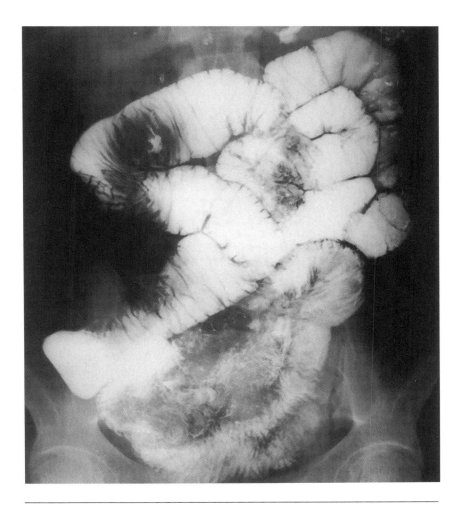

41a Name three radiological abnormalities seen on this barium follow-through of a patient under investigation for longstanding diarrhoea.

41b What are two possible diagnoses?

41c What complication has occurred?

41a   i) Small bowel dilatation, best seen in the mid and distal jejunum (normal calibre of mid small bowel is less than 3 cm), but normal small bowel folds.

      ii) Flocculation of the barium – areas where the barium has a coarse granular appearance (due to excess fluid in the bowel lumen).

      iii)Large filling defect in the barium column in the mid jejunum (to the right of L2).

41b   i) **Coeliac disease** – gluten-sensitive enteropathy.

      ii) **Tropical sprue**

41c   In this patient with longstanding coeliac disease, a **jejunal adenocarcinoma** has developed.

The radiological appearances of the small bowel in coeliac disease and tropical sprue are identical and closely relate to the clinical state of the patient. Those who are most severely ill show the most severe small bowel dilatation which reverses with treatment. Small bowel dilatation is seen in 70 – 95% of cases of untreated coeliac disease and is frequently associated with hyper-secretion related artifacts (break-up of the normal continual barium column and flocculation). Similar appearances may be seen in Whipple's disease, but there may be additional evidence of lymphadenopathy or bone changes.

A firm diagnosis depends on small bowel biopsy. Coeliac disease is associated with an increased incidence of gastrointestinal malignancy (lymphoma 8%, adenocarcinoma of the small bowel 6%, oesophageal and pharyngeal carcinoma).

Other causes of malabsorption with specific radiological features include jejunal diverticulosis, previous surgery, lymphoma and scleroderma.

CASE 42

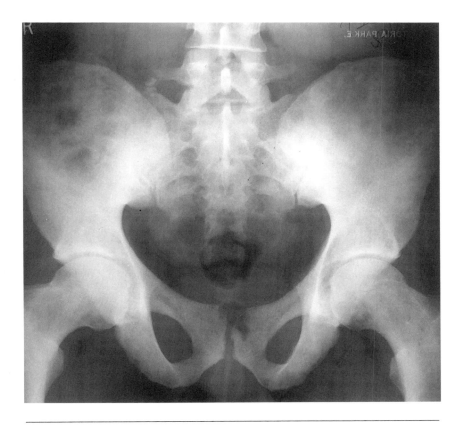

A pelvic X-ray of a 60-year-old male with anaemia.

42a   Describe two radiological abnormalities.

42b   What is the likely diagnosis?

42a   i) Diffuse increase in bone density (osteosclerosis) with lack of distinction between cortical and medullary bone.

ii) Splenomegaly (tip of spleen almost overlaps the left iliac crest).

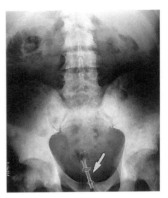

42b   **Myelosclerosis**
About half the patients with myelosclerosis have a widespread diffuse increase in bone density that primarily affects the spine, ribs and pelvis but may affect the whole skeleton. Uniform obliteration of the fine trabecular margins of ribs results in sclerosis resembling jail bars crossing the thorax. Extramedullary haematopoiesis causes massive splenomegaly.

Fig. 42A. Sclerotic bone metastases from prostatic carcinoma. Note the prostatic stent (arrow).

Other conditions causing a generalized increase in bone density include:

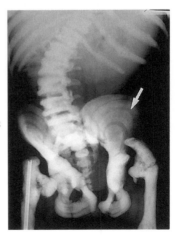

- Sclerosing bone metastases, particularly from prostate (Fig. 42A) or breast carcinoma.
- Paget's disease. Characteristic bone expansion and coarse trabeculation also present.
- Renal osteodystrophy.
- Fluorosis. Calcification of ligaments is also often present.
- Osteopetrosis (Fig. 42B). Rare hereditary bone dysplasia. The involved bones are dense but brittle and fractures are common. Characteristic 'bone within bone' appearance.
- Sickle cell disease. Additional features may include gallstones and step deformities in vertebral body endplates as well as avascular necrosis of femoral or humeral heads.

Fig. 42B. Osteopetrosis. Previous fractures, 'sandwich' lumbar vertebrae and 'bone within bone' appearances (arrow) are seen.

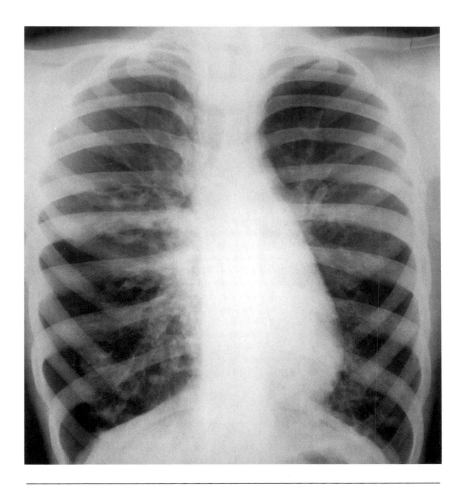

43   What is the likely cause of haemoptysis in this 50-year-old male?

43   **Bronchiectasis**
Multiple ring shadows are seen predominantly in the mid and lower zones, some of which contain air-fluid levels. Ring shadows represent dilated bronchi seen 'end on'. Bronchial wall thickening is also present.

Causes of bronchiectasis include:
- Childhood infections – especially measles and pertussis.
- Congenital structural defects.
  Kartagener's syndrome (Fig. 43A) – associated with immobile cilla, dextrocardia and absent frontal sinuses.
  Williams–Campbell syndrome.
- Immune deficiency states, e.g. hypogammaglobulinaemia.
- Secondary to bronchial obstruction – foreign body, neoplasm, mucous plugs (cystic fibrosis) and aspergillosis.

Thin section CT scanning is a more sensitive investigation for bronchiectasis and typically shows bronchi of greater calibre than their accompanying arteries.

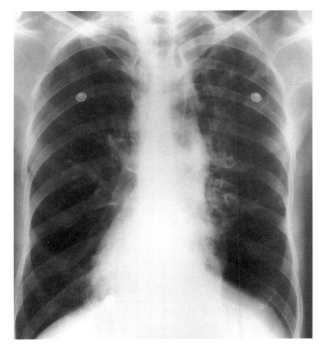

Fig. 43A. Kartagener's syndrome. Bronchiectasis and dextrocardia shown.

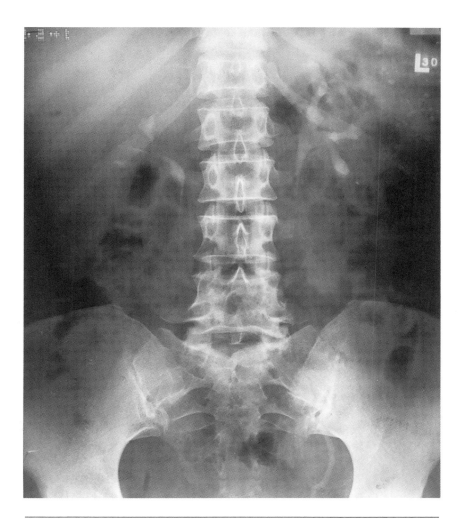

44a   Describe three radiological abnormalities seen on this IVU.

44b   What is the unifying diagnosis?

44a i) Multiple small calcific foci in the spleen, reflecting previous
        miliary disease.

ii) Irregularities of multiple calyces of the right kidney.

iii)Complete loss of the L4/L5 disc space due to a previous discitis.

44b **Tuberculosis (TB)**

The urogenital tract is the second most common site after the lung.
Evidence of previous TB on chest X-ray is seen in 10–15% of cases but less
than 5% have active pulmonary disease.

Extrarenal signs on the abdominal film include calcified granulomas in the
liver, spleen, lymph nodes and adrenal glands and paraspinal changes of TB
(discitis and psoas abscess).

Renal manifestations are unilateral in 75% of cases and include calyceal
deformities, stricture formation (pelvicalyceal system and ureter) and often
calcified masses. Autonephrectomy may occur (small shrunken, scarred,
non-functioning kidney ± dystrophic calcifications).

Vesical involvement leads to a reduction in bladder capacity. Prostatic,
epididymal and seminal vesicle calcification may also be seen.

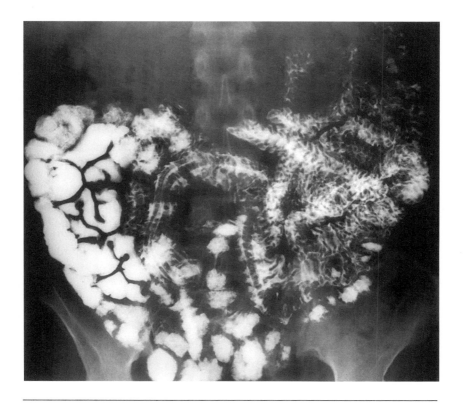

45   What is the cause of this lady's abdominal pain?

45   *Ascaris lumbricoides* (**roundworm**) **infestation in the small bowel.**

Roundworm infestation is common in tropical areas but may be seen in any part of the world. The adult worm appears as a tubular filling defect in the barium filled intestine. Within the tubular filling defect, a central thin thread of barium indicates that the worm has ingested some of the barium into its own alimentary canal. In children the worms may multiply forming conglomerate masses which may give rise to intestinal obstruction. Trapping of gas between these coiled clusters of worms may cause a 'whirled' appearance or so-called 'Medusa locks' – which may be seen on the plain film.

The tape worm (*Taenia solis*) may give a similar appearance but, unlike the roundworm, it has no alimentary canal and so cannot ingest the barium.

CASE 46

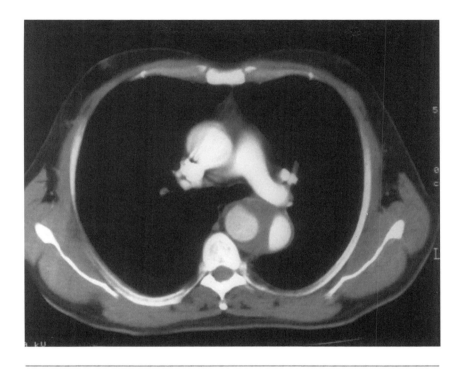

A CT scan of the thorax after intravenous contrast.

46   What is the diagnosis?

46   **Aortic dissection**

Two contrast filled channels are seen in the descending thoracic aorta, where there is normally only one. Note the differential flow in the true and false lumens (i.e. different densities) in this type B dissection (confined to the descending thoracic aorta).

Additional signs that may be seen are inward displacement of atherosclerotic plaque by 4–10 mm from the outer aortic contour, left pleural effusion and pericardial effusion (particularly if extending into the ascending aorta).

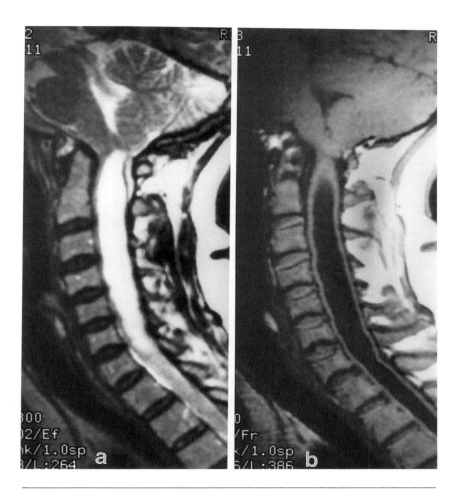

A sagittal MRI scan of the cervical spine, (a)T_2 and (b)T_1-weighted images.

47   What is the diagnosis?

47   Syringomyelia

A cystic cavity is seen within the cervical spinal cord which is itself expanded. The cavity has discrete, smooth, well-defined borders and a uniform signal intensity which is isointense with respect to CSF (i.e. high signal on the T_2-weighted image and low signal on the T_1-weighted image). It extends from C1 into the thoracic cord, but the lower limit is not shown on these images.

In syringomyelia the cervical cord is involved most often and is enlarged in about 80% of cases. A widened spinal canal may be seen on plain X-ray in 30%, but the condition is best demonstrated by MRI. Extension into the brain stem = syringobulbia.

Between 70–90% of cases of syringomyelia are associated with cerebellar ectopia (Arnold–Chiari malformation), the cerebellar tonsils usually lying at the level of C1 or between C1 and C2. Other than congenital causes, it may result from trauma, post-inflammation (e.g. infection, subarachnoid haemorrhage, surgery) and tumours.

Low signal may be seen within the cavity on T_2-weighted images due to CSF pulsations (flow–void phenomenon).

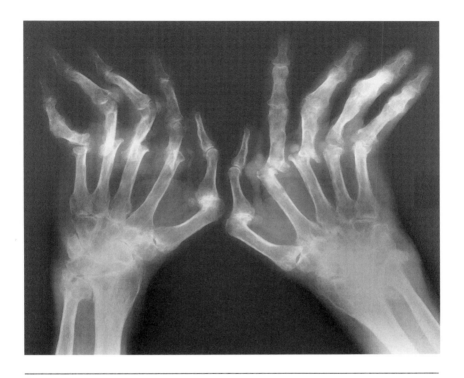

48a   Give three radiological abnormalities shown.

48b   What is the most likely diagnosis?

48a i) Bilateral, symmetrical, erosive polyarthritis predominantly
        affecting the metacarpophalangeal (MCP), proximal
        interphalangeal (PIP) and carpal joints.

      ii) At affected joints there is marked loss of joint space, bone
        resorption and soft tissue swelling. Subluxations are seen at the
        MCP joints, causing ulnar deviation.

      iii)Periarticular osteopaenia.

      iv)Erosion of the ulnar styloid bilaterally.

      v) Bony ankylosis of several PIP joints.

Other abnormalities that may be seen are 'swan-neck' deformities
(hyperextension at the PIP joint, fixed flexion deformity at the distal
interphalangeal [DIP] joint) and boutonnière deformities (fixed flexion at
the PIP joint with hyperextension at the DIP joint).

48b   Characteristic radiological appearances of **rheumatoid arthritis**.

Soft tissue swelling, joint space narrowing and periarticular erosions in
psoriatic disease may simulate rheumatoid arthritis but psoriasis usually
affects distal rather than proximal interphalangeal joints, is asymmetric and
causes little or no periarticular osteoporosis.

CASE 49

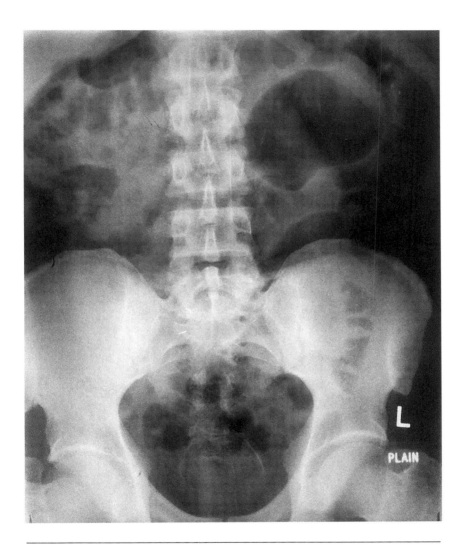

A 40-year-old male with haematuria.

49a   What abnormality is visible?

49b   What is the likely diagnosis?

49a   **Bladder wall calcification**

49b   **Urinary schistosomiasis**

Schistosomiasis is the commonest cause of bladder wall calcification worldwide and is the result of infestation by *Schistosoma haematobium*.

Thin, curvilinear calcification outlines a bladder of normal size and shape. Calcification may spread proximally to involve the distal ureters (appearing as two thin parallel lines) in 15%. Chronic infestation may be complicated by squamous cell carcinoma of the bladder.

Other causes of bladder wall calcification are:
*   Transitional and squamous cell carcinoma of the bladder. Radiographic incidence only 0.5%.
*   Tuberculosis. Rare and usually accompanied by calcification elsewhere in the urogenital tract. Unlike schistosomiasis the disease begins in the kidney and spreads distally.
*   Cyclophosphamide-induced cystitis.

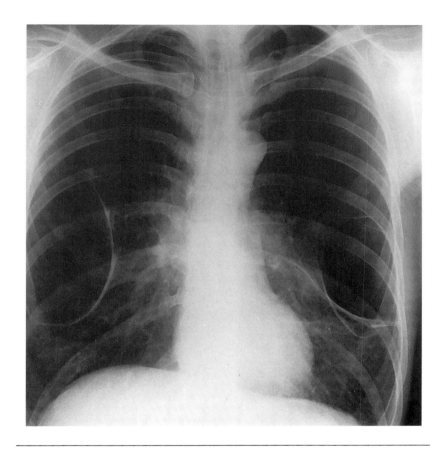

50   What is the diagnosis?

50 **Emphysema** – predominantly affecting the upper lobes (most common distribution and associated with smoking). Bullae are present in both lower zones.

The radiological findings ascribed to emphysema include:
- Hyperinflated lungs.
  The most reliable criterion is probably that of a low, flat diaphragm. In general a right hemidiaphragm that is at or below the anterior end of the seventh rib in the midclavicular line can be considered low.
- A reduction in the number and size of pulmonary vessels and their branches, particularly in the outer aspect of the lung.
- Avascular areas with curvilinear hair line margins, i.e. bullae.
- Secondary, right-sided cardiac enlargement.

When other conditions occur in emphysematous lungs, the radiological appearances are modified, e.g. with heart failure the oedema may spare emphysematous lung. CT scanning is a more sensitive way of detecting emphysema than plain chest radiography.

In alpha-1 antitrypsin deficiency (Fig. 50A), the striking feature of the emphysematous changes is its lower zone predominance and bullae are not a major feature.

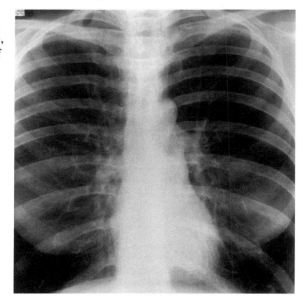

Fig. 50A. A female patient with alpha-1 antitrypsin deficiency.

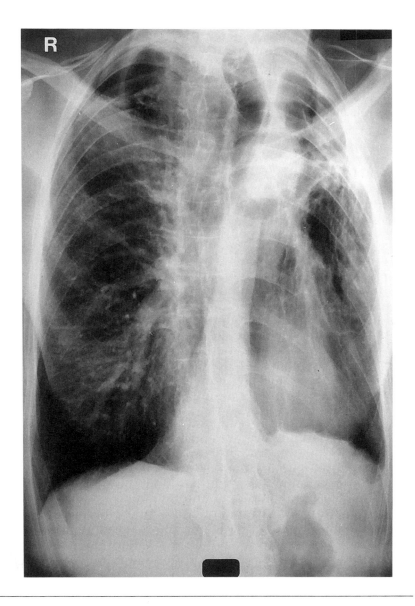

51   What two separate radiological abnormalities are seen on this chest
      radiograph of a young male patient?

51 i) Cavitating fibrosis predominantly affecting the left upper lobe, with parenchymal distortion and elevation of the left hilum.

ii) Lumbar spine syndesmophytes and 'bamboo' spine.

Appearances are compatible with a patient with **ankylosing spondylitis**. Mycetoma formation may occur within the lung cavities.

Other causes of upper lobe fibrosis are:

*   Tuberculosis – calcification is frequent.
*   Sarcoidosis – no calcification ± 'eggshell' calcification of lymph nodes.
*   Chronic extrinsic allergic alveolitis.
*   Radiotherapy – no calcification. May have mastectomy or radiation osteonecrosis of ribs or clavicles. The fibrosis tends to have well-defined straight borders corresponding to the radiation field.

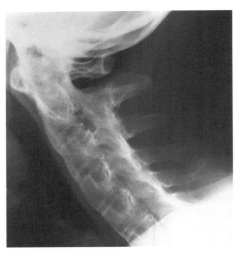

Fig. 51A. Fused cervical spine in ankylosing spondylitis.

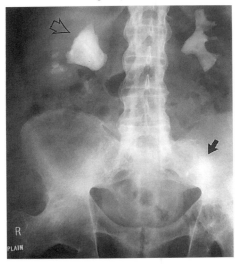

Fig. 51B. 'Bamboo' spine and ankylosed sacroiliac joints (arrow) in ankylosing spondylitis plus incidental bilateral staghorn renal calculi (open arrow). Note changes are also seen in both hips.

CASE 52

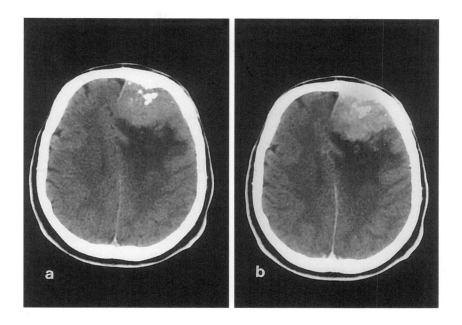

52a   Describe four radiological signs shown on these CT brain scans
        (a) Pre- and (b) Post-intravenous contrast.

52b   What is the most likely diagnosis?

52a i) A well defined left frontal, broad-based mass containing calcifications and of slightly increased density on the unenhanced scan relative to normal brain.

ii) Enhancement of the mass following contrast.

iii)Thickening and sclerosis of the adjacent skull vault.

iv)Low attenuation surrounding the mass in the left frontal lobe, consistent with cerebral oedema, plus some midline shift from left to right.

52b **Left frontal meningioma**

Meningiomas are solid, well-circumscribed, generally benign tumours that arise from the meninges, projecting inward from the dura and indenting and compressing the underlying brain.

These extracerebral tumours account for approximately 20% of adult brain tumours. Frequent sites of origin include the frontal and parietal convexities and parasagittal regions as well as the sphenoid wing, olfactory groove and suprasellar regions.

Multiple meningiomas occur in 6–9% and are associated with neurofibromatosis.

Typical CT radiological features of a meningioma include hyperdensity (± calcifications in 15%) pre-contrast (in 95%), adjacent bone thickening (90%) and striking homogeneous enhancement of the tumour mass.

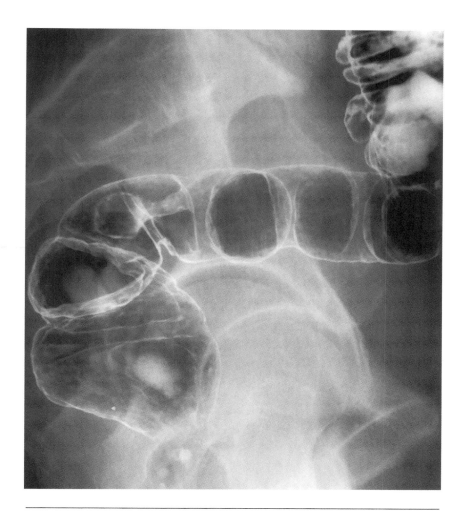

53   What is the likely diagnosis?

53   A large colonic polyp (proven to be neoplastic at biopsy)

A large, solitary, pedunculated polyp is seen in the distal sigmoid colon on this lateral view of the rectum from a barium enema series. Ninety-three per cent of colorectal carcinomas arise from adenomatous polyps and most commonly occur in the sigmoid colon (20–37%).

The malignant potential of a colonic polyp depends upon its size and degree of cellular dysplasia. Polyps measuring 5–9 mm are most likely to be adenomatous and have a 1% probability of containing invasive malignancy. Polyps measuring 1–2 cm in diameter have a 4–10% incidence of malignancy. Polyps more than 2 cm in diameter have a 20–40% incidence of malignancy.

Other signs of malignancy include irregular or lobulated surface, retraction (puckering) of the colonic wall and interval growth or change in shape. Double contrast barium enemas detect 82–98% of polyps greater than 1 cm in size.

Colonic tumours may have various appearances which include a discrete polyp, annular constriction or saddle lesion.

There is a 1% risk of multiple synchronous colonic tumours and a 3% risk of metachronous tumours.

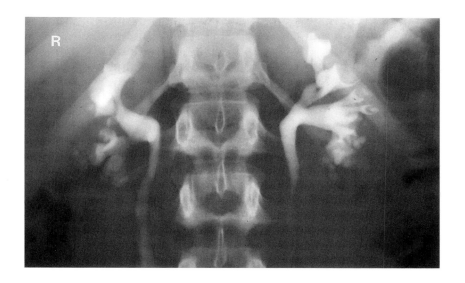

54   What is the diagnosis in this 45-year-old patient with a history of chronic back pain?

54   **Renal papillary necrosis** – probably secondary to analgesics. Renal papillary necrosis is bilateral in 85% of cases with multiple papillae affected. Papillae show varying degrees of deformity which vary from long and thin to short and bulbous and includes cavity formation. A 'ball and cup' type appearance may be seen (as in the left kidney in this case).

If total sloughing ensues the sloughed papillary tissue may:
- Fragment and be passed in the urine.
- Cause ureteric obstruction.
- Remain free in a calyx.
- Remain in the renal pelvis and calcify.

Calyces appear club-shaped or round following total sloughing of a papilla.

The causes of renal papillary necrosis include:
*A*nalgesics – phenacetin and aspirin
*D*iabetes mellitus
*I*nfants in shock
*P*yelonephritis   }   *ADIPOSE* is a useful mnemonic
*O*bstruction
*S*ickle cell disease
*E*thanol

However, diabetes, analgesics and sickle cell anaemia are the most frequent causes.

CASE 55

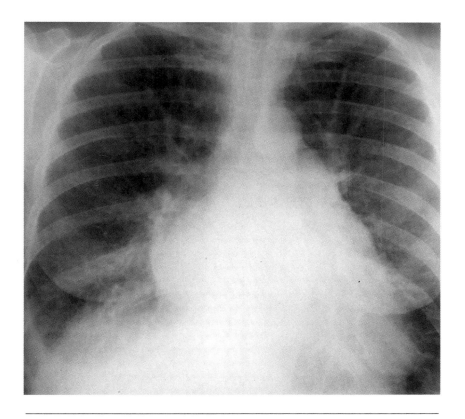

55a   Describe three radiological abnormalities shown.

55b   What is the diagnosis?

55a   The radiological abnormalities shown include:
- Cardiomegaly with left atrial enlargement.
- Redistribution of blood flow (due to pulmonary venous hypertension). The upper zone vessels are similar in size to lower zone vessels and normally the lower zone vessels are larger.
- Enlargement of the pulmonary trunk – suggesting pulmonary arterial hypertension.
- Bilateral basal, peripheral septal lines (Kerley B lines).

55b   **Mixed mitral valve disease**

Signs of left atrial enlargement on the chest radiograph are:
- Prominent left atrial appendage (an additional bulge is seen below the pulmonary trunk).
- Double right heart border.
- Splaying of the carina and elevated left main bronchus.

Septal lines are linear densities, 1–3 cm long, less than 1 mm thick, extending from and perpendicular to the pleural surface. Best seen in the costophrenic angles. Septal lines are most often seen in interstitial pulmonary oedema when they are due to fluid collecting in the interlobular septae. Other causes are lymphangitis carcinomatosa (Fig. 55A), sarcoidosis and silicosis. If transient or rapid in development, they are virtually pathognomic of left ventricular failure.

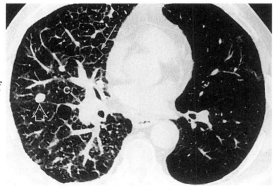

Fig. 55A. High resolution CT scan showing unilateral thickened interlobular septae (arrow) (corresponding to septal lines on the chest radiograph), typical of lymphangitis carcinomatosa. Note the right hilar bronchogenic carcinoma (C) and metastasis (open arrow).

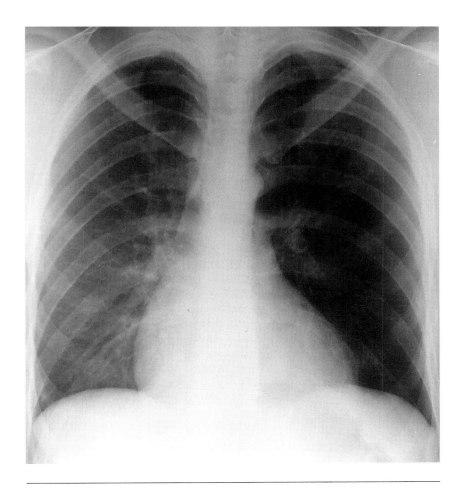

56a   Describe two abnormalities on this expiratory chest X-ray of an asymptomatic male.

56b   What is the likely diagnosis?

56a   i) Hypertransradiant left hemithorax with evidence of air trapping on this expiratory radiograph.

          ii) Small left hilum and reduced left pulmonary vasculature.

56b   **Macleod's (Swyer–James) syndrome**

Probably due to a childhood viral illness causing an obliterative bronchiolitis. On an inspiratory radiograph the abnormal, hypertransradiant hemithorax is generally of normal or reduced volume. Air trapping is seen on expiration.

It can be difficult in the presence of unequal lucency on a chest X-ray to decide which is the abnormal side. **A useful rule is:**
- If vascularity is decreased, the lung is abnormal.
- If vascularity is normal or increased, the lung is probably normal.

Causes of a unilateral hypertransradiant hemithorax include:
- Patient rotation (commonest cause). Check that the trachea is midway between the medial ends of the clavicles.
- Chest wall abnormalities, including mastectomy, Poland's syndrome (unilateral congenital absence of pectoral muscles) and poliomyelitis. Note that the vasculature will be normal.
- Pneumothorax: look for the lung edge.
- Pulmonary embolus: to a major pulmonary artery.
- Lung: obstructive emphysema (e.g. an inhaled foreign body), congenital lobar emphysema (most commonly the left upper lobe), unilateral bullae and Macleod's syndrome.

NB   Exclude contralateral increased density, e.g. pleural effusion in a supine patient, or pleural thickening.

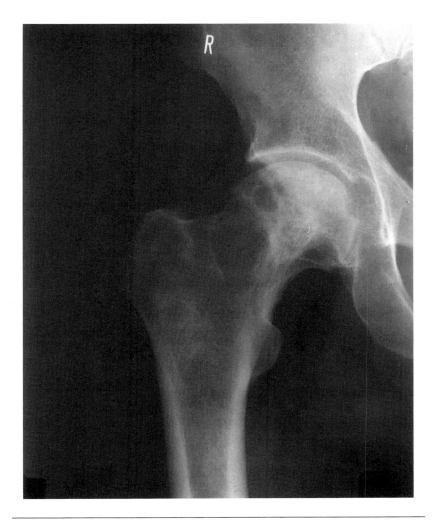

This radiograph was obtained during a routine occupational health examination of a 45-year-old male.

57a   Describe the radiological abnormalities.

57b   What is the diagnosis?

57c   Suggest two possible causes.

57a Patchy sclerosis throughout the flattened femoral head and narrowing of the joint space.

57b **Avascular necrosis (AVN) of the femoral head**

57c i) Caisson disease (dysbaric disorders) – as in this case. Exposure to high pressure environments, as occurs in deep sea diving or tunnel construction may subsequently lead to osteonecrosis.

ii) Other causes of avascular necrosis include: sickle cell disease, steroids, radiation, trauma, idiopathic (Perthes' disease), collagen vascular disorders, infection and alcoholism.

The hip is the most common site involved in AVN, the hallmark of which is increased bone density at an otherwise normal joint. Radiological changes may take several weeks to appear and, in addition, include subchondral lucency, sclerosis, collapse of the articular surface and joint fragmentation.

MRI plays a valuable role in the early diagnosis of AVN (Fig. 57A) and is more sensitive than radionuclide scans.

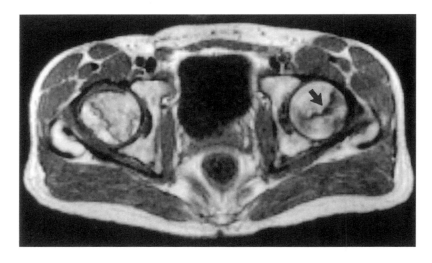

Fig. 57A. MRI scan (axial) T_1-weighted image showing typical findings of AVN affecting both hips. Note the serpiginous cleft of low signal intensity (arrow) giving the appearance of 'tennis balls'.

CASE 58

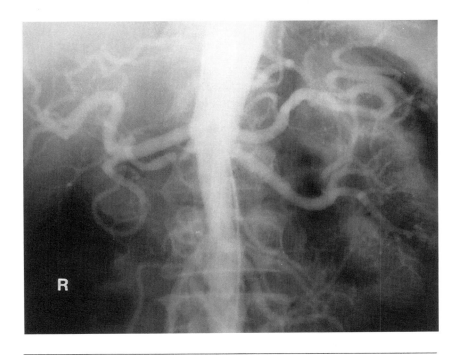

58   What is the likely cause of hypertension in this 55-year-old man?

58   **Right renal artery stenosis** – due to arteriosclerosis. The right kidney is smaller than the left and there is a tight stenosis of the proximal 1 cm of the right renal artery.

Arteriosclerosis is responsible for two-thirds of renovascular causes of hypertension and typically affects the proximal 2 cm of the renal artery. It is more common in males.

This is in contrast to fibromuscular dysplasia, responsible for one-third of renovascular causes of hypertension, which mainly affects women under the age of 40 and occurs in the mid and distal renal artery, sparing the proximal third of the main renal artery in 98% of cases. It is bilateral in 60% of cases and, if alternating areas of stenoses and dilatations are present (60–70%), a string of beads' appearance occurs.

The signs of unilateral renal artery stenosis on IVU are:
*   A small smooth kidney.
*   Unilateral delay of one minute or more in the appearance of opacified calyces.
*   Increased density of opacified calyces.
*   Ureteric notching by collateral vessels.

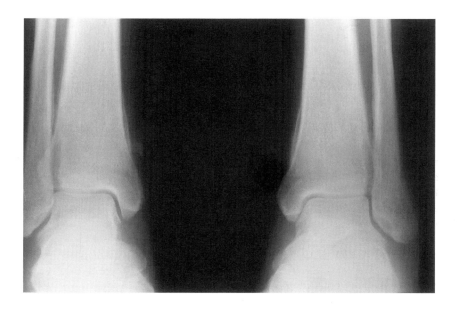

59a   What is the cause of the abnormality seen on this X-ray of the ankles?

59b   List three diseases with which this condition is associated.

59a **Hypertrophic osteoarthropathy** (HOA): an exuberant periosteal reaction of the tibia and fibula.

59b i) Pleural fibroma (local benign mesothelioma).

ii) Bronchogenic carcinoma.

iii) Less commonly: congenital cardiac disease, intrathoracic sepsis, inflammatory bowel disease and liver disease.

Periosteal proliferation of new bone, at first smooth and then rough and undulating is seen earliest along the distal third of the radius and ulna, then the distal tibia and fibula. Distal phalanges and the axial skeleton are rarely affected.

Radiologically, soft tissue swelling may be seen over distal phalanges if clubbing is present, but the underlying bone is normal and erosions do not occur. In the long bones, periostitis affects the distal diaphyses, but the bone ends are not involved. It causes a painful symmetrical arthropathy.

The vast majority of cases are associated with bronchogenic carcinoma, up to 12% of which have HOA, with the exception of oat cell carcinomas.

Of the benign causes, the highest incidence is found with pleural fibroma (Fig. 59A).

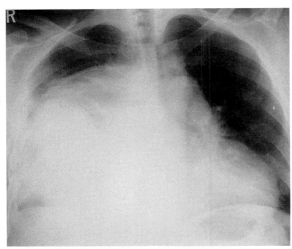

Fig. 59 A Large right pleural fibroma, causing mediastinal shift to the left.

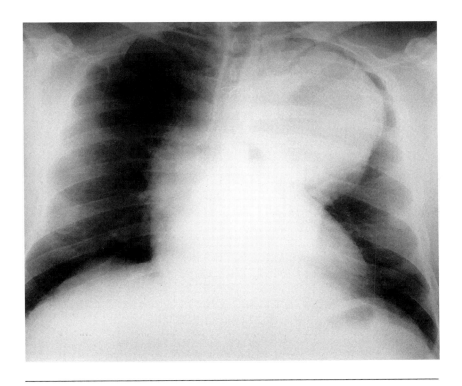

60   What is the likely diagnosis in this tall thin young male?

60   **Aortic aneurysm**
      There is marked enlargement of the aortic arch on the chest
      radiograph of this patient with Marfan's syndrome. The large
      superior mediastinal mass is continuous with the descending aorta
      inferiorly and appearances are consistent with an aortic aneurysm
      (confirmed on CT – Fig. 60A). Median sternotomy wires reflect a
      previous attempt at repair.

Other causes of an enlarged aortic arch are hypertension (which by itself
only leads to slight unfolding, with left ventricular enlargement), aortic
incompetence (prominent ascending aorta) and aortic stenosis (post-stenotic
dilatation ± aortic valve calcification).

Unfolding of the aorta often gives the impression of an enlarged aortic arch
and is a common finding in the elderly.

Aetiologies of thoracic aortic aneurysm include:
*   Atherosclerosis – prominent calcification.
*   Trauma.
*   Infection, e.g. syphilitic aortitis, subacute bacterial endocarditis.
*   Intrinsic abnormality, e.g. Marfan's syndrome.

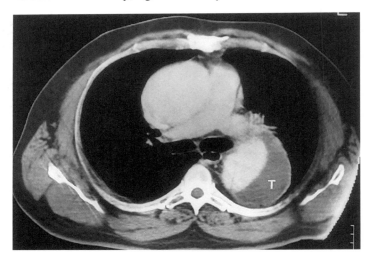

Fig. 60A. Contrast-enhanced CT of the thorax showing a large aortic
aneurysm involving both the ascending and descending thoracic aorta.
Note the eccentric thrombus (T) in the descending aorta.

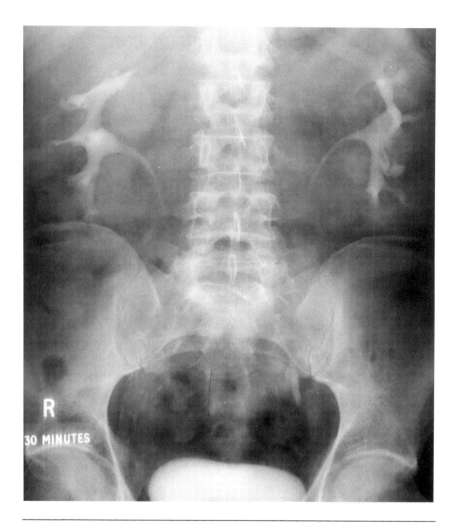

61   What is the cause of this patient's hypertension?

61   **Polycystic kidney disease**
The IVU shows that both kidneys are enlarged (normal renal size approximates to the length of three vertebral bodies and their discs) and there is marked distortion of the collecting systems caused by the multiple cysts.

Associations include:
*   Cysts in the liver (25–50%) and pancreas (9%).
*   Saccular berry aneurysms of cerebral arteries (10–30%).

This appearance is easily distinguished from other causes of large kidneys including renal infiltration (lymphoma, amyloid), urine outflow obstruction (hydronephrosis), interstitial fluid accumulation (renal vein thrombosis, acute tubular necrosis) and proliferative disorders (acute glomerulonephritis).

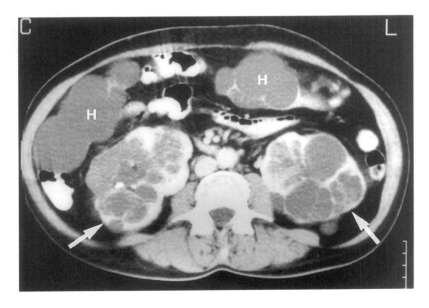

Fig. 61A. Enhanced CT scan of the abdomen showing polycystic kidneys (arrows) and multiple hepatic cysts (H).

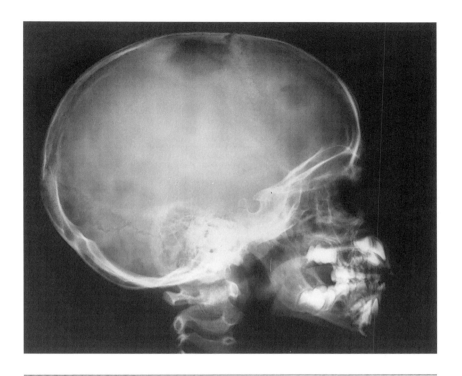

62a   What abnormality is seen on this skull X-ray of a 25-year-old patient with a chronic condition?

62b   What is the probable diagnosis?

62a   Two, large well-defined areas of bony destruction are present (one near the vertex and the other in the frontal region). Both have bevelled edges. The frontal lesion has a sclerotic rim (seen in spontaneous healing or following treatment).

62b   **Langerhans cell histiocytosis** (known previously as histiocytosis X)

Other radiological abnormalities in this condition include:
- Skeleton – 50–75% have solitary lesions. Long bones, pelvis, skull and flat bones are the most common sites involved. Punched out lucencies in the skull vault may coalesce to give a 'geographical skull' and involvement of the mandible may produce 'floating teeth'.
- Lung involvement in <10% is associated with a worse prognosis. Honeycomb lung, often with spontaneous pneumothoraces. Mid and upper zones are predominantly affected and lung volume is normal or increased (a useful sign).

CASE 63

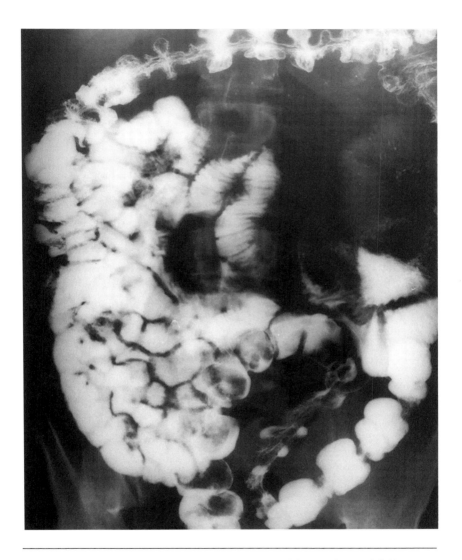

63a   What radiological abnormality is seen on this small bowel follow-through examination?

63b   What is the differential diagnosis for this appearance?

63a   There are multiple strictures in the small bowel of varying length (Fig. 63A shows an enlargement of a segment of jejunum) – due to **lymphoma** in this case.

63b   The differential diagnosis for multiple small bowel strictures includes:

- Crohn's disease – indistinguishable from lymphoma, although there is usually additional evidence of altered mucosal pattern and ulceration (either longitudinal or transverse fissure ulcers or aphthoid ulcers). Strictures may be short or long, single or multiple.
- Tumours – including lymphoma (generally secondary to contiguous spread from lymph nodes), carcinoid and metastases.
- Tuberculosis – may be radiologically identical to Crohn's disease. Terminal ileum, caecum and ascending colon are often affected in continuity. Generally the stenotic lesions are shorter and the caecum more contracted than in Crohn's disease.
- Adhesions – history useful. Angulation of bowel which remains constant in site. Normal mucosal pattern.
- Radiation enteritis – typically in the distal jejunum and ileum. Absence of ulceration, cobble stoning and asymmetry differentiates it from Crohn's disease.
- Infarction – progression is rapid, strictures tend to be long and ulcers are rare.

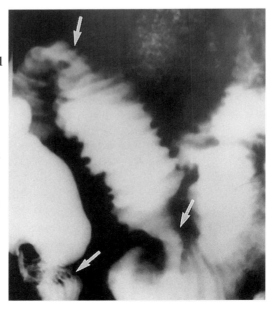

Fig. 63A. Magnified view of small bowel strictures (arrowed).

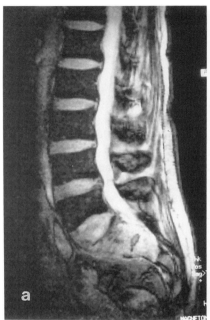 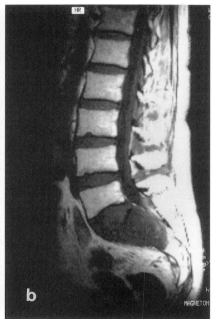

A 36-year-old female with breast carcinoma.

64   What radiological abnormality is seen on these sagittal (a) T_2-
        weighted and (b) T_1-weighted images of the lumbosacral spine?

64   **A large sacral metastatic deposit**
The bone marrow here shows marked alteration, with low signal on
T_1-weighted images and high signal on T_2-weighted images and there
is extension into the L5/S1 disc space and sacral canal.
The vertebral bodies otherwise appear normal.

In adults, approximately 50% of all spine metastases arise from breast, lung
or prostate cancer. All vertebral levels can be involved, although the lower
thoracic and lumbar spine are the most frequently affected sites. Imaging
findings – most metastases are osteolytic, although breast and prostate
cancer can cause sclerotic lesions. Pedicle destruction is the most common
plain film finding. Other frequent abnormalities include multifocal lytic
vertebral body lesions, pathologic compression fractures and paraspinous
soft tissue masses.

Bone scintigraphy is sensitive in the detection of metastases; only a 5–10%
change in lesion to normal bone area is needed (which compares to 40–50%
destruction needed for detection on plain films). However, bone scans are
non-specific and may also be falsely negative in multiple myeloma in which
case radiographic examination is more sensitive for detecting osteolytic
lesions.

MRI is even more sensitive than bone scintigraphy in detecting vertebral
metastases and exquisitely delineates cord compression, epidural and
paraspinous soft tissue involvement. The most common pattern is multifocal
lytic lesions, characterized by low signal intensity on T_1 and high signal
intensity on T_2-weighted sequences.

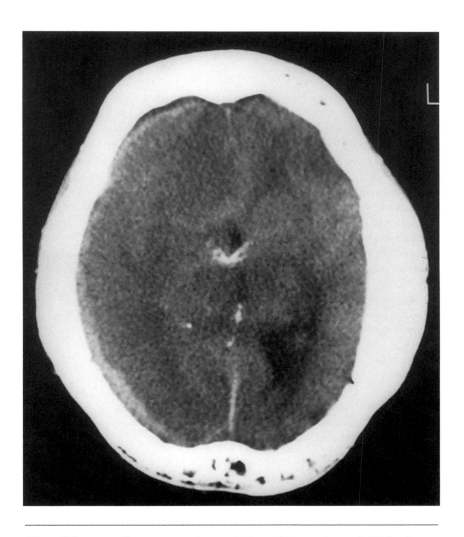

65   What two diagnoses can be made from this unenhanced CT head
      scan of a 70-year-old male?

65   i) **Acute right-sided subdural haematoma**, causing mass effect, compression of the right lateral ventricle and shift of the midline from right to left.

ii) **Paget's disease**. Note the abnormally thickened skull vault.

Subdural haematomas arise as a result of rupture of bridging veins and are seen predominantly in infants and the elderly and may be bilateral (25% in adults). 40% of small subdural haematomas are missed.

Characteristically, there is an extra-axial, peripheral, high attenuation crescenteric-shaped fluid collection. Concave inner margin and convex outer margin, following the normal contours of the skull vault, to be distinguished from the lenticular shape of an extradural collection. Extension of blood into the interhemispheric fissure also indicates a subdural location.

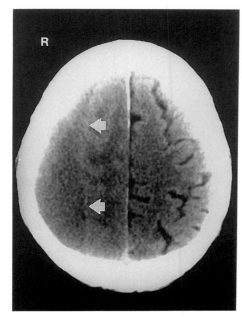

Density of collection changes with time:

Hyperdense	(< 1 week)
Isodense	(1–3 weeks) –
see Fig. 65A	
Hypodense	(3–4 weeks)

In most cases the subdural haematoma is accompanied by ipsilateral cerebral oedema and mass displacement.

Fig. 65A. Isodense right subdural haematoma (the inner margins are arrowed). The skull vault appears artifactually thickened at this level, due to a partial volume effect from the vertex.

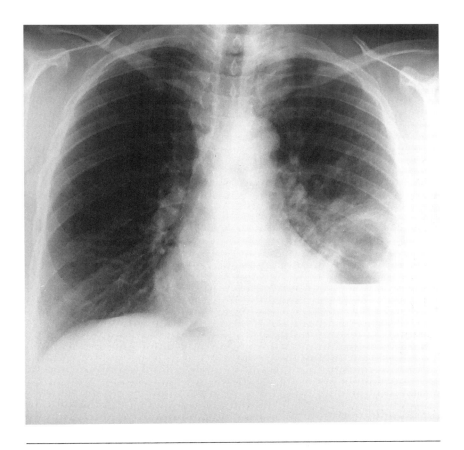

66 What pulmonary complication has occurred in this patient who has recently had a general anaesthetic?

66   A lung abscess

An ill-defined rounded mass is seen in the left lower zone in an area of consolidation (note the lack of visualization of the left hemidiaphragm). The opacity contains an air-fluid level.

On the lateral view (Fig. 66A), the air-fluid level is of a similar length indicating that the mass is spherical and most likely therefore to be a lung abscess.

The CT scan (Fig. 66B) shows the abscess more clearly. It has irregular, thick walls and note the acute angle that its walls make with the adjacent pleura (for the differentiation from empyema see Case 85).
Causes of lung abscesses include:

- *Staphylococcus aureus* – thick walled, with an irregular lining. No lobar predilection. Associated with effusion and empyema. More common in children.
- *Klebsiella pneumoniae* – has a similar appearance, but favours the upper lobes and usually single.
- Tuberculosis – thick walled and smooth. Upper lobes and apical segments of lower lobes favoured. Usually surrounded by consolidation.
- Aspiration – a foreign body, e.g. tooth may be apparent.
- Others – Gram-negative organisms, nocardiosis, aspergillosis, actinomycosis, amoebiasis and hydatid.

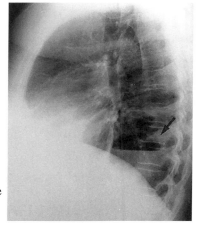

Fig. 66A. Lung abscess (lateral view), projected posteriorly over the dorsal spine (arrow).

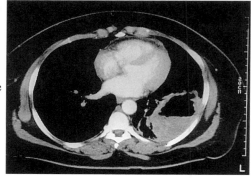

Fig. 66B. Contrast-enhanced CT scan – left lower lobe abscess with a thick, irregular wall.

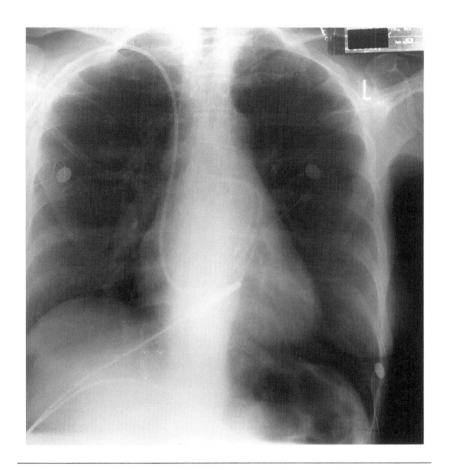

A 35-year-old female with acute onset of dyspnoea.

67a   What does the chest radiograph show?

67b   What is the diagnosis?

67a   The left lung appears oligaemic with few vascular markings and absence of the left main pulmonary artery. ECG leads, oxygen tubing and a catheter whose tip lies in the pulmonary outflow tract are noted.

67b   A large left main pulmonary embolus

The diagnosis is confirmed by the pulmonary angiogram (Fig. 67A). Multiple filling defects consistent with emboli are also seen on the right side.

Pulmonary emboli are more frequent in the lower zones and are often multiple (65%). Pulmonary infarction will only occur in approximately one third of these patients.

Chest radiographs are frequently normal (>30%). Abnormal findings include diaphragmatic elevation, abrupt tapering of a pulmonary artery, secondary local oligaemia and linear atelectasis. Parenchymal consolidation occurs with infarction and is generally basal and associated with a small pleural effusion. Cavitation may occur. Chronic pulmonary emboli lead to pulmonary hypertension.

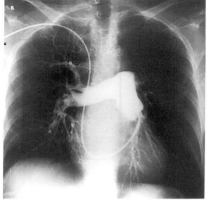

Fig. 67A. Pulmonary angiogram – large embolus in the left main pulmonary artery and multiple small right pulmonary emboli.

Ventilation/perfusion isotope scanning is a useful diagnostic method and a normal perfusion scan virtually excludes a pulmonary embolus. Recently, spiral CT angiography has been shown to successfully demonstrate emboli in the main, and segmental pulmonary arteries, but is unreliable for subsegmental disease (Fig. 67B).

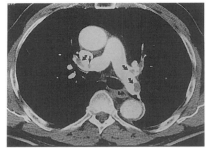

Fig. 67B. Spiral CT scan showing multiple pulmonary emboli as filling defects in the main pulmonary arteries (arrows).

CASE 68

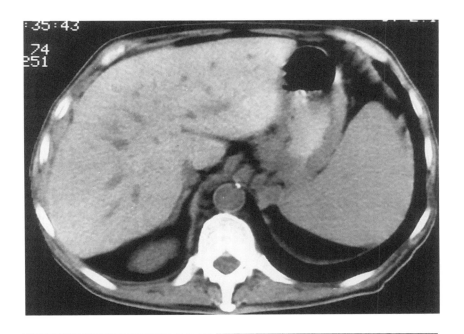

An unenhanced CT scan of the upper abdomen in a 40-year-old male with arthralgia and diabetes.

68a   What radiological abnormality is shown?

68b   What is the likely diagnosis?

68a   A generalized increase in liver density. Note the increased
       discrepancy in attenuation between liver and spleen. Also,
       intrahepatic vessels, not normally visualized on non-enhanced scans,
       stand out as low density against the high density background.
       Liver density is similar to that of the oral contrast (iodine containing)
       in the adjacent stomach.

68b   **Haemochromatosis**

A diffuse increase in liver density pre-intravenous contrast may be due to:
*   Haemochromatosis – there may be additional features of cirrhosis,
    portal hypertension or an associated hepatoma.
*   Iron overload – e.g. from a large number of blood transfusions.
*   Amiodarone treatment – contains iodine.
*   'Thorotrast' deposition – generalized (often inhomogeneous)
    increased density of the liver and spleen is caused by this previously
    used contrast agent. This alpha-emitting radionuclide has been
    associated with the development of hepatobiliary carcinoma and
    leukaemia.
*   Gold therapy for rheumatoid arthritis.

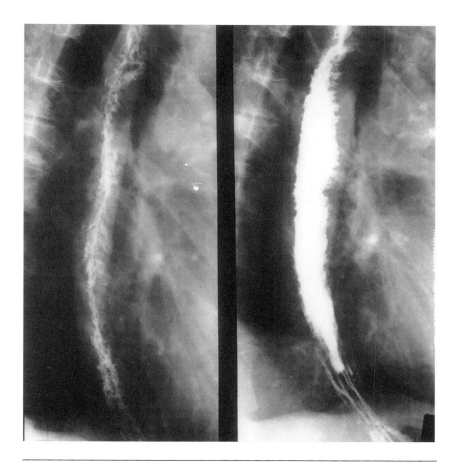

69a   What does the barium swallow of this 40-year-old patient, who had a previous renal transplant, show?

69b   What is the likely cause of his dysphagia?

69a   Extensive oesophageal mucosal irregularity with ulceration, producing a 'shaggy' appearance of the oesophagus in profile.

69b   **Oesophageal moniliasis**

This tends to occur in patients debilitated by malignant disease, diabetes, alcohol, renal failure or, immunosuppressant, cytotoxic or steroid therapy. Identical appearances are produced by infection with *Herpes simplex*. However, gastro-oesophageal reflux remains the most common cause of oesophagitis in which case a hiatus hernia is usually present.

Differentiation from oesophageal varices, which produce serpiginous filling defects in the barium pool is generally easy (see Case 38).

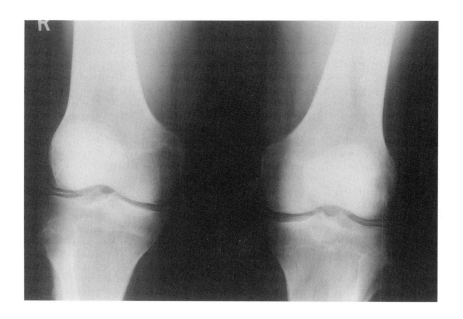

70a   What abnormality is shown?

70b   Name three causes of this appearance.

70a **Chondrocalcinosis** – calcification of articular cartilage.

70b Chondrocalcinosis may be seen in:
*W*ilson's disease
*H*yperparathyroidism, haemochromatosis
*I*diopathic (ageing)
*P*seudogout (calcium pyrophosphate dihydrate deposition disease)
*A*cromegaly
*D*iabetes mellitus
*O*chronosis
*G*out
Mnemonic – *WHIP A DOG*

Chondrocalcinosis can occur in any joint but tends to affect the medial and lateral compartments of the knee, the triangular fibrocartilage of the wrist and the symphysis pubis. It is most commonly due to pseudogout.

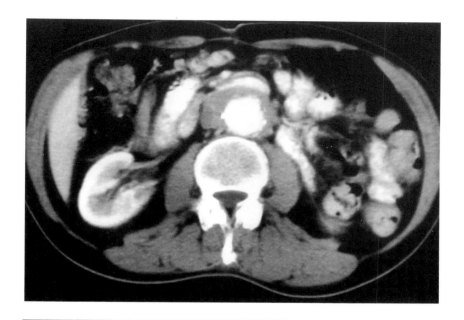

71a   What abnormality is seen on this upper abdominal CT scan (with intravenous and oral contrast) of a 40-year-old male with back pain?

71b   What is the diagnosis?

71c   What other radiological features may be seen on IVU in this condition?

71a   Periaortic mass of attenuation similar to muscle.

71b   **Retroperitoneal fibrosis**

71c   i) Medial deviation of ureters in their middle third, typically
       bilateral, which is more significant if there is a right-angled step in
       the course of the ureter rather than a gentle drift. The position of
       the ureters is, however, frequently normal.

       ii) Ureteric obstruction of varying severity (75% bilateral) and
       usually at the L4/L5 level. Hydronephrosis.

Causes of retroperitoneal fibrosis include:
- Retroperitoneal malignancy (8%) – lymphoma and metastases
  especially from breast and colon.
- Inflammatory conditions – Crohn's disease, diverticular disease,
  pancreatitis.
- Drugs (12%) – methysergide, phenacetin, hydralazine.
- Aortic aneurysm.
- Retroperitoneal trauma and surgery.
- Idiopathic – 75% of all cases may be due to an immune reaction to
  atheromatous material in the aorta. May respond to corticosteroids.

Despite apparent ureteric obstruction, the ureters are often easily
catheterized retrogradely, e.g. for stent placement.

CASE 72

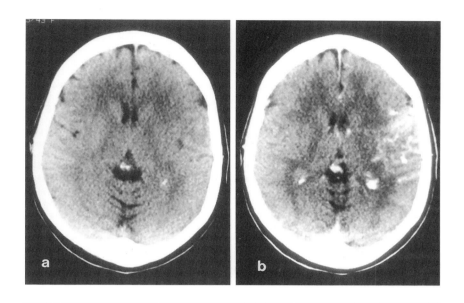

A CT head scan– (a) Pre- and (b) Post-intravenous contrast.

72   What is the likely cause of seizures in this 40-year-old man?

72   **Arteriovenous malformation** (AVM) – a congenital abnormality
      most often supratentorial (90%) and commonly in the parietal lobe.

      No definite abnormality is seen on the pre-contrast scan. Following
      contrast, large tortuous high attenuation structures are seen in the left
      parietal lobe (representing serpiginous, dilated vessels), lack of mass
      effect or oedema.

An unruptured arteriovenous malformation may appear normal or only
subtly abnormal on unenhanced scans since the abnormal vessels are usually
only slightly hyperdense with respect to the brain and therefore difficult to
identify.

In some cases, calcification suggests the presence of a malformation and
may be seen on a skull film (15–30%) as may prominent vascular grooves
due to the dilated feeding vessels. AVM may be complicated by
haemorrhage with a 2% risk per year of recurrent bleeding.

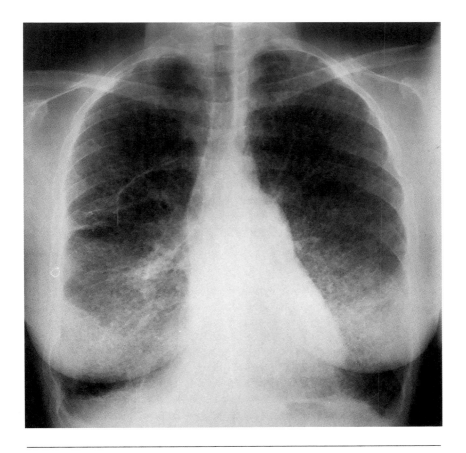

73a   Describe the radiological abnormalities seen in this 25-year-old female.

73b   Give two possible diagnoses.

73a   There is a coarse, reticular, interstitial pattern which has a mid and
       lower zone predominance. The lung volumes are, however, increased.
       Evidence of a previous lung biopsy in the right mid-zone (line of
       sutures).

73b   i) **Lymphangioleiomyomatosis**

       ii) **Tuberous sclerosis**

Virtually all interstitial lung disorders are associated with progressive loss in
volume (e.g. Case 17) unlike the following four conditions which are
associated with a progressive <u>increase</u> in lung volume:

- Lymphangioleiomyomatosis: exclusively affects women of child-
  bearing age. Characterized by an excessive accumulation of muscle
  in relation to extrapulmonary lymphatics. Recurrent pneumothorax
  (40%), large chylothorax (50–75%) and eventual honeycombing are
  seen.
- Tuberous sclerosis: radiographic appearances identical to
  lymphangiomyomatosis, including a high incidence of recurrent
  pneumothorax. However, chylothorax is unusual and other features,
  including epilepsy and adenoma sebaceum, are often apparent.
- Langerhans cell histiocytosis: similar radiographic appearances
  (occurring in <10% of patients) often with a nodular component, but
  differing in that there is generally an upper lobe predominance.
  Recurrent pneumothorax is seen in 25% but pleural effusion is
  uncommon. Ninety per cent of patients are smokers.
- Neurofibromatosis: as well as the typical interstitial lung changes
  seen in 20% of patients and favouring the lower zones, other features
  are generally present, including rib notching, twisted 'ribbon' ribs,
  cutaneous tumours (appearing as nodules on the chest radiograph)
  and kyphoscoliosis.

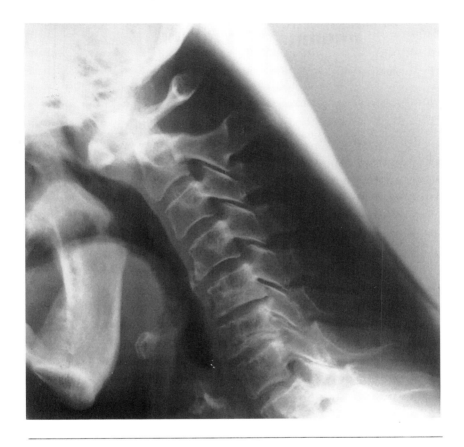

A routine pre-operative lateral cervical spine X-ray.

74a   What abnormality is shown?

74b   Name three conditions in which this complication can occur.

74a **Atlanto-axial subluxation** – diagnosed when the distance between the posterior aspect of the anterior arch of the atlas and the anterior aspect of the odontoid process exceeds 3 mm in adults or 5 mm in children.

74b Atlanto-axial subluxation may be seen in:
- Rheumatoid arthritis: in 20–25% of patients with severe disease. Associated erosion of the odontoid process, as in this case, is often seen.
- Psoriatic arthropathy: in 45% of patients with spondylitis.
- Ankylosing spondylitis: in 2% of cases.
- Juvenile chronic arthritis: most commonly in seropositive juvenile onset adult rheumatoid arthritis.
- Systemic lupus erythematosus.
- Congenital disorders, e.g. Down's syndrome.
- Associated with a retropharyngeal abscess in a child.

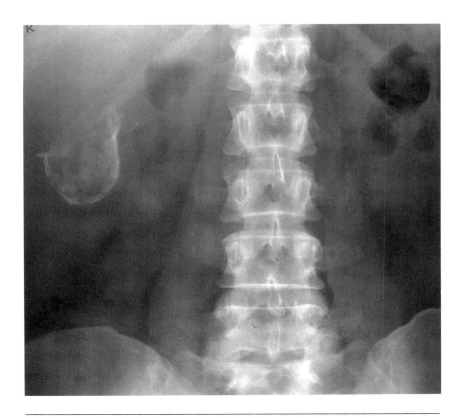

75   What radiological abnormality is shown?

75   Calcification of the gall bladder wall (**Porcelain gall bladder**).

Mural calcification around the perimeter of the gall bladder is found in
0.6–0.8% of cholecystectomy patients and is associated with chronic
inflammation and hence the presence of gallstones (in 90%). The cystic duct
is usually blocked. There is an increased incidence of carcinoma of the gall
bladder.

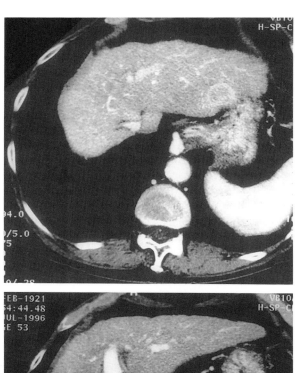

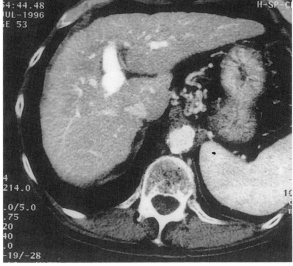

76a   Describe three radiological abnormalities on this contrast-enhanced CT scan through the upper abdomen of a 50-year-old alcoholic.

76b   What is the likely diagnosis?

76a   i) Irregular surface of the liver – compatible with cirrhosis.

ii) A solitary ring-enhancing rounded mass in the left lobe of the liver (upper image).

iii)Serpiginous opacities anterior to the aorta along the lesser curve of the stomach are varices.

Further images revealed splenomegaly (> 12 cm length) and no additional hepatic lesions. No ascites.

76b   **Cirrhosis with portal hypertension and hepatocellular carcinoma (HCC).**

HCC is associated with cirrhosis (most often due to alcoholism, hepatitis B virus or haemochromatosis) in 60–90% of cases. Approximately 5% of patients with alcoholic cirrhosis develop HCC which is most commonly a solitary lesion, showing enhancement during the arterial phase on CT scanning.

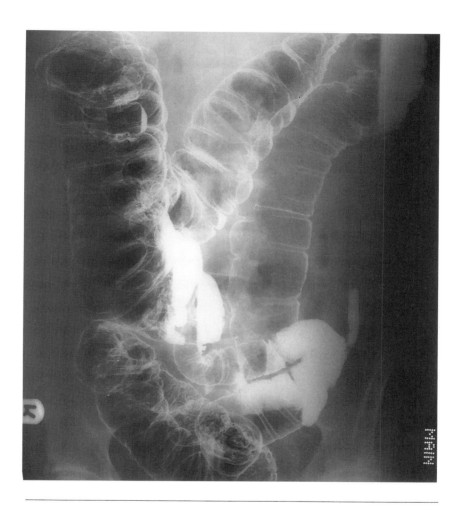

77   What radiological abnormality is seen on this barium enema of a
      patient with chronic abdominal pain?

77   A **Meckel's diverticulum** – arising from the terminal ileum
      (projected over the left ilium).

Meckel's diverticulum occurs in 2% of subjects (most in children < 10 years
of age) on the anti-mesenteric side of the ileum within 100 cm of the
ileocaecal valve. It is the most frequent congenital anomaly of the intestinal
tract; an outpouching of the rudimentary omphali-mesenteric duct.

Presentation varies:
- Gastrointestinal bleeding due to ulceration of heterotopic gastric
  mucosa present in 30% of patients; (60% in symptomatic children).
- Acute diverticulitis.
- Intestinal obstruction secondary to intussusception/fibrous
  bands/volvulus.
- Chronic abdominal pain.

Diagnosis may be made by an isotopic method following injection of
Tc 99 pertechnetate which is taken up strongly by ectopic gastric mucosa
(sensitivity drops after adolescence), or by barium enema with reflux of
barium into the terminal ileum. It is seldom recognized on small bowel
enema. Extremely rarely, it may appear as a large gas-filled viscus with a
fluid level on the horizontal ray film.

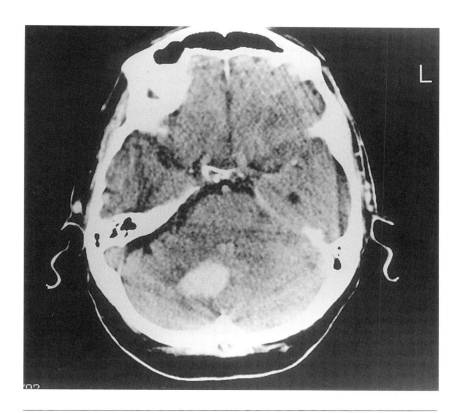

78   What complication has occurred in this 65-year-old hypertensive man who collapsed suddenly?

78   **Acute cerebellar haemorrhage** (right hemisphere) with extension of high density material (blood) into the fourth ventricle.

In the majority of cases intracerebral haemorrhage occurs as a result of hypertension. Less frequent causes include arteriovenous malformation, aneurysm, trauma, vasculitis, anticoagulant therapy, tumour haemorrhage (e.g. melanoma metastases, glioma) and haemorrhagic infarctions.

Blood can penetrate into the ventricles or subarachnoid spaces and give rise to hydrocephalus.

The fresh haematoma is a sharply demarcated, round or oval focus of homogeneously increased attenuation. The indirect signs of a space-occupying lesion are often present. The density of a haematoma decreases slowly, and is isodense with normal brain after 3–6 weeks, typically resorbing from outside towards the centre.

Other causes of hyperdense cerebral masses on CT:
- Neoplasms: meningiomas (95%), lymphoma, metastases (30%) – particularly from melanoma, adenocarcinoma, renal cell carcinoma, bronchogenic carcinoma, glioma (10%) – most glioblastomas show mixed attenuation, ependymoma, medulloblastoma (80%), pituitary adenoma (25%), acoustic neuroma.
- Aneurysm.
- Colloid cyst (50%) – occurs in young adults, anterior to the third ventricle. Well-defined.

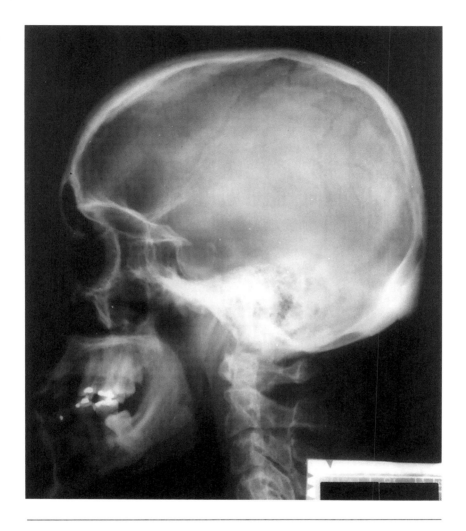

79a   Describe the two radiological abnormalities shown.

79b   What is the diagnosis?

79a i) Enlargement and erosion of the pituitary fossa.
ii) Prognathism (increased angle of mandible).
iii)Enlarged paranasal air sinuses and mastoids.
iv)Enlargement of the occipital protuberance.

79b **Acromegaly**

Other effects of excessive growth hormone on the mature skeleton include:
* Vertebrae: an increase in AP and transverse dimensions with posterior scalloping in 30%. Kyphosis.
* Hands: 'spade-like' with broadening of the fingers (Fig. 79A) and terminal tufts ('oak trees'). Widening of metacarpophalangeal joints due to cartilage hypertrophy.
* Joints: premature osteoarthritis and chondrocalcinosis.
* Soft tissues: increased heel pad thickness (> 25 mm).

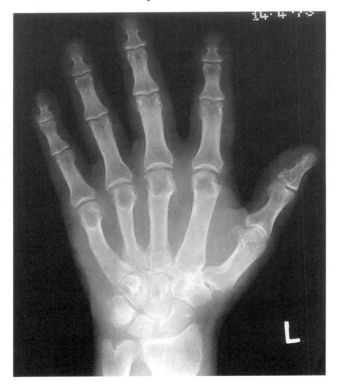

Fig. 79A. Acromegaly 'spade-like' hand.

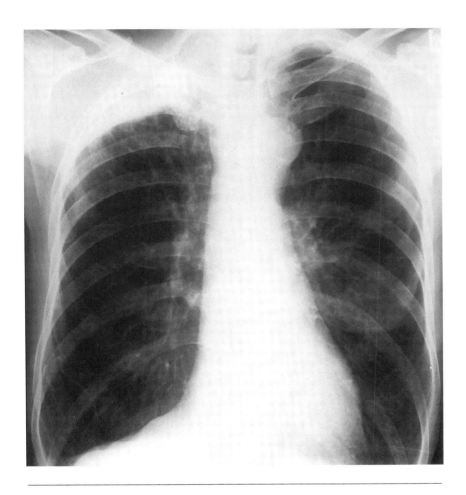

80a   Describe two abnormalities shown.

80b   What is the likely diagnosis in this 65-year-old patient with a painful right shoulder?

80a   i) A right apical mass.

ii) Destruction of the right second rib.

80b   An apical bronchogenic carcinoma (**Pancoast or superior sulcus tumour**).

Pancoast's original description included ipsilateral Horner's syndrome, due to invasion of the sympathetic chain, and local destruction of bone by the tumour, which may be of any cell type.

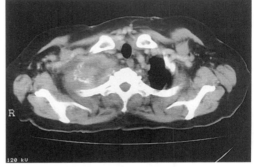

Fig. 80A. CT scan – right Pancoast's tumour.

Radiographically, the tumours appear as a mass in 50–75% of cases and as an apical cap (resembling pleural thickening) in the remainder. Bone destruction is seen in one third of cases in the adjacent ribs or spine.

CT can be helpful (Fig. 80A) for showing the full extent of the tumour, particularly chest wall invasion, although MRI provides superior information in this respect due to its multiplanar capability.

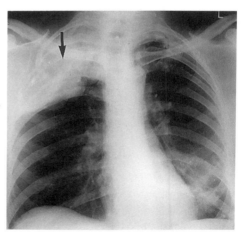

Another cause of apical opacification is plombage (Fig. 80B). The lucite balls have smooth lower margins and there is often evidence of previous tuberculous infection at the other lung apex.

Fig. 80B. CXR. Plombage (arrow). Evidence of previous TB at the left apex; calcification, pleural thickening and upper lobe fibrosis with elevation of the left hilum. In addition there is acute, left basal consolidation due to a bacterial pneumonia.

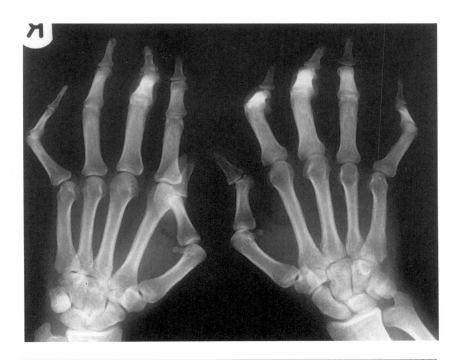

81a   Describe two radiological abnormalities.

81b   What is the likely diagnosis in this 30-year-old female with a chronic condition?

81a   i) Subluxations and malalignment of joints in the absence of erosions. Note the boutonnière deformities of both thumbs.

ii) Sclerosis of several middle phalanges.

81b   **Systemic lupus erythematosus (SLE)**
A non-erosive deforming polyarthropathy may be seen in SLE and after subsidence of frequent severe attacks of rheumatic fever (Jacoud's arthropathy).

Other causes of phalangeal sclerosis are:
*   Normal variant – 10% of the population.
*   Rheumatoid arthritis – most commonly in association with erosive arthropathy.
*   Scleroderma – in addition to soft tissue calcification, tuft resorption and joint erosions.
*   Sarcoidosis – a lacy reticular pattern is often associated.

CASE 82

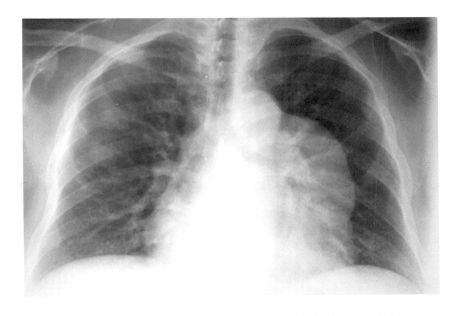

A chest radiograph of a 55-year-old male.

82a   Describe the radiological abnormality.

82b   What is the likely diagnosis?

82a   There is a large, lobulated soft tissue density mass projecting to the left of the mediastinum. The descending thoracic aorta, aortic arch and left main pulmonary artery can still be seen clearly, placing the mass in the anterior mediastinum. No associated calcifications or pleural disease.

82b   **Thymoma**

Thymomas are unusual in patients under the age of 20 and occur in 10–17% of patients with myasthenia gravis and are usually benign. They are round or oval and smooth or lobulated. They may contain nodular or rim calcification or fat. They usually arise near the junction of the heart and great vessels (see lateral view, Fig. 82A) and may protrude to one or both sides of the mediastinum.

A few are situated more inferiorly, adjacent to the left or right borders of the heart. They are best evaluated radiologically with CT.

Invasive thymomas (30% of cases) show spread beyond the capsule and metastases may be seen.

Other causes of anterior mediastinal masses are:
*   Lymphoma – enlargement of anterior mediastinal and retrosternal lymph nodes. There is often symmetric widening of the superior mediastinum on frontal views.
*   Teratoma – usually larger than thymomas. Calcification and fragments of bone or teeth may be seen. More than 80% are benign.
*   Retrosternal goitre – goitre extends into the superior mediastinum in 1–3% of cases and continuity with cervical soft tissues is visible. The trachea may be displaced.

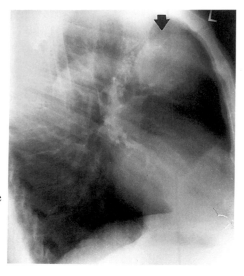

Fig. 82A. Lateral CXR. Thymoma (arrow).

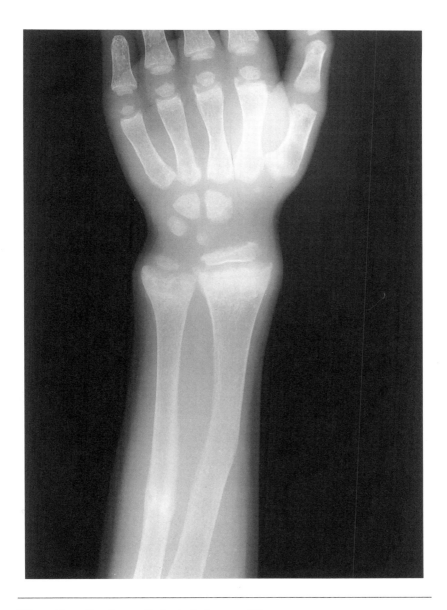

83a Describe four radiological abnormalities.

83b What is the likely diagnosis?

83a   i) Abnormal metaphyses, with cupping and fraying.

ii) Generalized osteopenia.

iii)Bowing deformities.

iv)Looser's zone (mid-shaft of ulna).

v) Soft tissue swelling around the wrist.

83b   **Rickets** (secondary to anticonvulsant medication).

Radiological features are due to non-calcification of recently formed osteoid and to the effects of stress on the weakened bone and are most obvious at the wrists and knees.

Looser's zones are demonstrated less often in children than in adults with osteomalacia. Other features (in addition to those above) are rickety rosary (cupping of the anterior ends of the ribs), scoliosis, skull bossing and retarded bone maturation and growth.

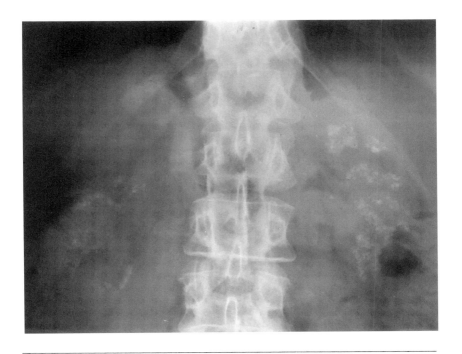

84   List three conditions in which this abnormality may be found.

84 i) **Hyperparathyroidism**

ii) **Renal tubular acidosis**

iii) **Medullary sponge kidney**

Renal parenchymal calcification (**nephrocalcinosis**) may be medullary – as in this case – or cortical.
- Medullary: the three causes above account for 70% of cases. Renal tubular acidosis is the commonest cause in children. Other causes include conditions producing hypercalcaemia or hypercalciuria, e.g. sarcoidosis, idiopathic hypercalciuria, hypervitaminosis D.
- Cortical: (5% of all nephrocalcinoses) – acute cortical necrosis, chronic glomerulonephritis and chronic transplant rejection.

Causes of more focal calcification include renal cell carcinoma, tuberculosis, hydatid disease and papillary necrosis.

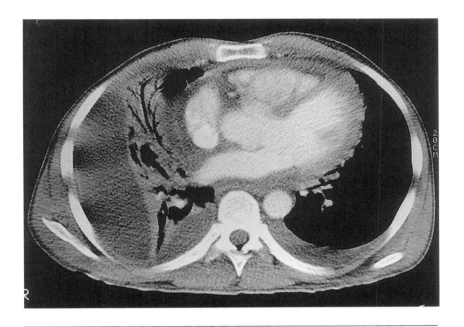

85   Describe four radiological abnormalities shown on this
      contrast-enhanced CT scan through the thorax.

85   i) **Pericardial effusion**: fluid density within the pericardial sac (compare with the normal pericardium in Fig. 66B).

ii) **Left pleural effusion**: fluid density within the dependent part of the left hemithorax.

iii)**Right middle and lower lobe consolidation**: (note the air bronchograms visible).

iv)A large right, lenticular shaped pleural collection (predominantly in the lateral part of the right hemithorax, i.e. non-dependent aspect) – likely to be an **empyema**.

The distinction between pulmonary abscess and loculated pleural fluid can be difficult, but has important therapeutic consequences. Empyema requires early tube drainage, whereas antibiotics are given as first-line treatment in most cases of pulmonary abscess.

Features that may help differentiate between abscess and empyema are:
- Shape: loculated collections of pleural fluid tend to be based on the parietal pleura and are lenticular shaped or oval. If an air-fluid level is present, it will therefore be substantially longer on one view than in the other on the chest films. Abscesses tend to be spherical.
  In empyema the angle formed at the interface with the chest wall is obtuse compared with the acute angle more commonly associated with abscesses.
- Wall: the walls of an empyema are formed by thickened pleura and tend to be of uniform thickness and smooth ('split pleura sign'). The thickened pleura may enhance. The wall of an abscess is more irregular and tends to be thicker than in empyema and may contain dots of air.
- Adjacent lung: lung adjacent to an empyema is often compressed, unlike with abscesses. Adjacent pneumonia is unhelpful as it may be associated with both.

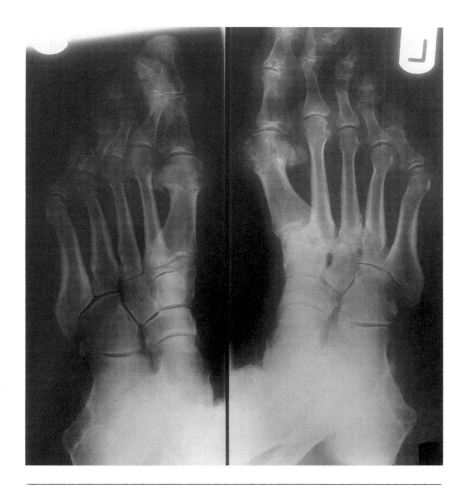

86a   What does this X-ray of both feet show in this 50-year-old man with swollen, painful toes?

86b   What is the likely diagnosis?

86a   Asymmetrical soft tissue swellings around the first metatarsophalangeal and interphalangeal joints associated with asymmetrical 'punched out' joint erosions at the joint margins (mostly set back from the articular surface). There is preservation of joint space and no apparent osteoporosis.

86b   The distribution of affected joints and type of erosions favours **gout**.

The first metatarsophalangeal joint is the most common joint affected in gout (called 'podagra') and the classic history is that of recurrent attacks becoming more severe, frequent and polyarticular.

Radiological features are typically seen late (generally more than six years after the first attack) and include soft tissue swelling and 'punched out' erosions which start near joint margins and have a classic overhanging margin in up to 40% and a sclerotic margin. Chronic tophaceous gout reveals eccentric soft tissue masses in a periarticular location (which rarely calcify).

Cartilage destruction (and hence joint space narrowing) is late and chondrocalcinosis occurs in 5% of cases.

The distribution of the arthropathy is usually asymmetric. The differential diagnosis includes rheumatoid arthritis which typically has joint space narrowing and osteoporosis and less well-defined erosions and psoriasis which has a predilection for the interphalangeal joints and does not have erosions that are this sharply defined.

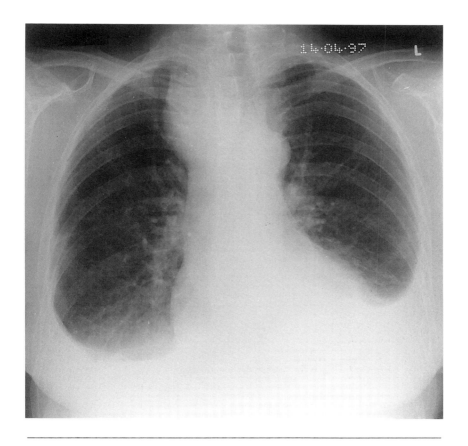

87   Describe three radiological abnormalities in this patient who has recently had an operation.

87   i) **Bilateral pleural effusions.**

      ii) **Median sternotomy wires** (recent coronary artery bypass grafting).

      iii)**A large right superior mediastinal mass**, continuous with the soft tissues of the neck and associated with tracheal shift to the left. No associated calcifications or hilar lymphadenopathy.

Appearances consistent with a **goitre**.

Of those goitres which have an intrathoracic component, 80% are located in the anterior mediastinum. Focal calcifications are common.

Anterior goitres typically displace the trachea posteriorly and laterally.

CASE 88

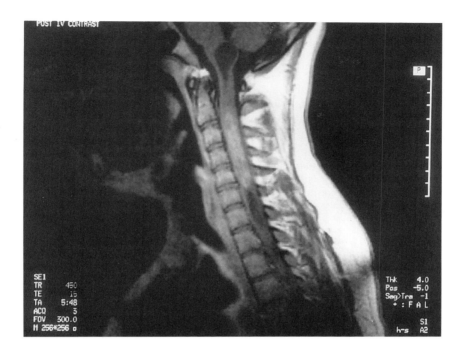

POST IV CONTRAST

SE1
TR 450
TE 15
TA 5:48
ACQ 3
FOV 300.0
H 256*256 o

Thk 4.0
Pos -5.0
Seg>Tra -1
÷ : F A L

SI
h-s A2

88a   Describe two radiological abnormalities shown on this T_1-weighted, enhanced, sagittal MRI scan of the neck.

88b   What is a likely diagnosis?

88a i) Focal expansion of the cervical spinal cord (C1–C6) by a
heterogeneously enhancing intramedullary lesion.

ii) A surrounding syrinx.

88b Appearances are those of an **intramedullary tumour**, most likely to
be a **glioma** (in this case an astrocytoma).

Mass lesions in the spinal canal are classified as extradural, intradural and
intramedullary in location.

- Extradural mass:
  Prolapsed or sequestered intervertebral disc
  Metastases
  Neurofibroma
  Neuroblastoma
  Meningioma
  Haematoma
  Abscess
  Arachnoid cyst

- Intradural mass:
  Meningioma
  Neurofibroma
  Metastases
  Subdural empyema

- Intramedullary mass:
  Ependymoma (65%) – commonest in the conus and the lumbar region.
  Astrocytoma (25%) – commonest in the cervical region. Appearance
  is similar to ependymoma
  Oligodendroglioma
  Metastases – with lung carcinoma as the most common primary
  Lipoma – common in conus
  Haematoma.

Following contrast there is striking enhancement of most intramedullary
neoplasms on both CT and MRI, although lesions are much better defined
on MRI.

NB The figures in brackets refer to the percentage of all intramedullary tumours.

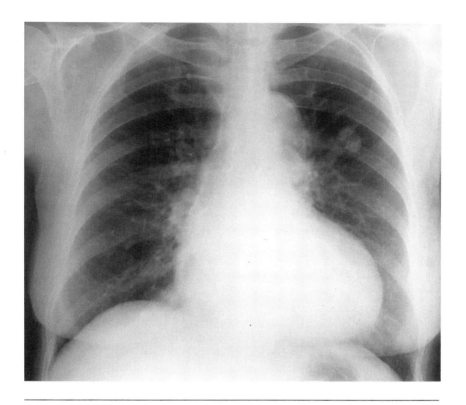

89a   Describe the radiological abnormality shown.

89b   What is the likely diagnosis in this patient with epistaxis and telangiectasia of the skin?

89a   There is a sharply defined, lobulated, solitary, oval mass in the left upper zone with a band shadow connecting it to the left hilum.

89b   Typical appearances of a **pulmonary arteriovenous malformation (AVM)** – with the band shadow representing the feeding artery and vein. The history suggests that the patient may have Osler–Weber–Rendu syndrome with which the majority of pulmonary AVMs are associated and in which case they tend to be multiple.

The differential diagnosis includes other causes of solitary pulmonary nodules:
- Granuloma: secondary to tuberculosis/histoplasmosis. Well defined and commonly calcified and the most common lung mass.
- Malignant neoplasm: bronchogenic carcinoma (accounts for less than 15% of all solitary pulmonary nodules at age 40) and calcification is very rare, metastases (25% are solitary) and alveolar cell carcinoma.
- Benign neoplasm: adenoma (90% occur around the hilum) and hamartoma (may have 'popcorn' calcification and usually within 2 cm of the pleura).
- Infections: pneumonia, hydatid, abscess.
- Congenital: sequestration and bronchogenic cyst.
- Vascular: haematoma and pulmonary infarction.

Features that may help differentiate include:
- Spiculations – strongly suggestive of primary malignancy (90% of irregular, spiculated lesions are malignant), whereas 80% of sharply marginated lesions are benign.
- Calcifications – most suggestive of granuloma.
- Change in size with time – a rapid increase in size suggests malignancy.
- A vessel leading to a mass indicates an AVM or pulmonary varix.

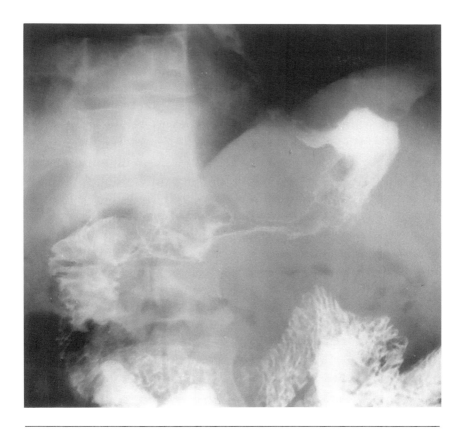

90a   What radiological abnormality is shown on this small bowel follow-through of a 70-year-old male with weight loss?

90b   Suggest a likely diagnosis.

90a   Diffuse, irregular narrowing and contraction of the stomach, particularly in the antrum and body regions.

90b   **Gastric carcinoma** (linitis plastica).

An identical appearance (of linitis plastica) can also be caused by:
- Lymphoma.
- Metastases (especially breast).
- Local invasion from pancreatic carcinoma.
- Corrosive ingestion.
- Radiotherapy.
- Crohn's disease.

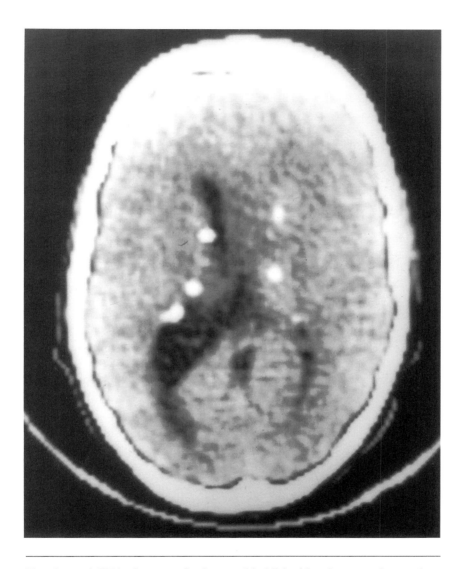

Unenhanced CT brain scan of a 4-year-old child with seizures and mental retardation.

91a   Describe the radiological abnormality shown.

91b   What other radiological features are seen in this condition?

91a   Multiple high attenuation (calcified) subependymal nodules are seen lining the lateral ventricles characteristic of **tuberous sclerosis**.

91b   Central nervous system:
   i) Cortical hamartomas: non-calcified, non-enhancing hypodense brain lesions.

   ii) Cerebral neoplasms: an enhancing mass typically near the foramen of Munro (giant cell astrocytoma).

Kidneys
*   Angiomyolipomas: in 40–80% of patients. Usually multiple and bilateral, the tumours contain fat.
*   Multiple renal cysts.
Skeleton – asymptomatic lesions
*   Irregular periosteal reaction.
*   Patchy sclerotic lesions.
Lungs
*   CXR: non-specific coarse generalized reticulonodular shadowing which progresses to honeycombing. The lungs, however, are of normal/large volume.
Heart
*   Cardiac rhabdomyomas.

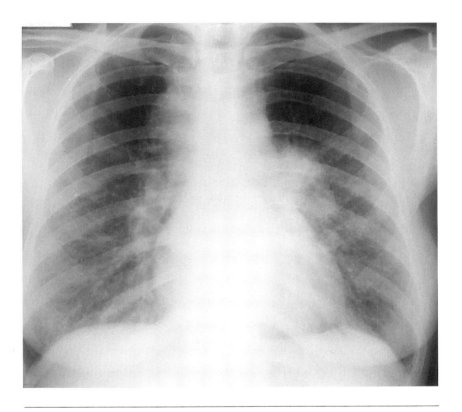

92   What is the likely diagnosis in this 25-year-old female with a history
      of night sweats and weight loss?

92   **Lymphoma**
The chest radiograph shows asymmetrical mediastinal and hilar
lymphadenopathy. Subcarinal lymphadenopathy is indicated by loss
of visualization of the azygo-oesophageal line (compare with Case
29, where the line can be clearly seen through the cardiac silhouette).
The lungs appear clear.

Intrathoracic lymphadenopathy is the most common manifestation of
lymphoma in the thorax and is more common in Hodgkin's disease. Nodal
involvement tends to be bilateral and asymmetrical and most commonly
involves anterior mediastinal nodes (refer to Case 29 for a discussion on
patterns of mediastinal lymphadenopathy in other conditions). Nodes show a
rapid response to radiotherapy and 'eggshell' calcification of lymph nodes
may be observed one to nine years after radiotherapy.

Lung involvement is very unusual without lymphadenopathy.

Causes of 'eggshell' nodal calcification include:
- Sarcoidosis: calcification of lymph nodes occurs in approximately
  5% of patients.
- Lymphoma following radiotherapy.
- Silicosis: seen in approximately 5% of patients. Lungs show multiple
  small nodular shadows.
- Coal-miners' pneumoconiosis: only occurs in 1% of cases.
  Associated pulmonary changes include miliary shadowing or massive
  shadows.

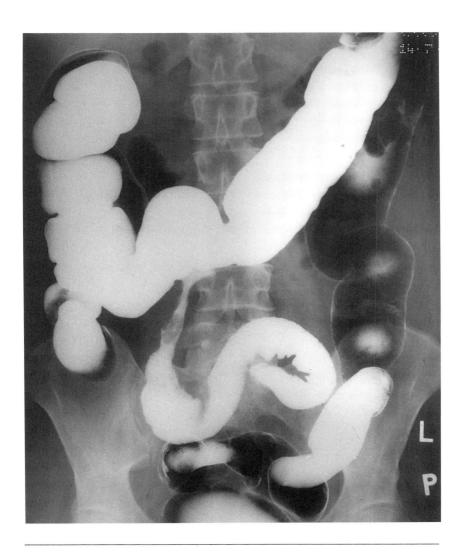

93   What is the likely diagnosis?

93   **Crohn's colitis**
The double contrast barium enema shows an abnormal appearance of
the terminal ileum, which is narrowed and irregular, typical of
Crohn's disease (an appearance termed the 'string sign of Kantor').
Normal right sacroiliac joint and lumbar spine. No evidence of a
colonic carcinoma.

Other radiological abnormalities that may be
seen in Crohn's disease are strictures which
may be single or multiple. Asymmetrical
involvement and skip lesions are
characteristic. Disease predominates on the
mesenteric border. Ulceration of various
degrees (Fig. 93A), with the terminal ileum
the commonest site. Complications include
fistulas, toxic megacolon, carcinoma (less
common than in ulcerative colitis),
lymphoma, gallstones, sclerosing cholangitis
and arthritis.

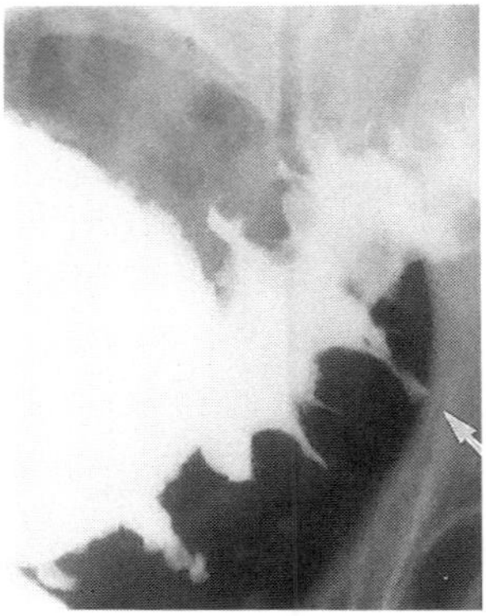

Other conditions affecting the terminal
ileum are:

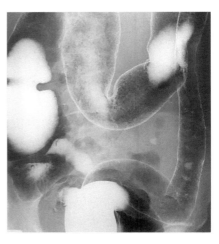

Fig. 93A. Rose-Thorn ulcers
(arrow).

*   Ulcerative colitis: 10% of
    those with total colitis have
    'backwash' ileitis for up to
    25 cm. No ulcers (Fig. 93B).
*   Tuberculosis (TB): can look
    identical to Crohn's disease,
    but predominantly it involves
    the caecum. Less than 50%
    have pulmonary TB.
*   Lymphoma: may mimic
    Crohn's disease, but often
    additional signs are present.
*   Less common causes include
    carcinoid, metastases,
    ischaemia (rare site) and
    radiation enteritis.

Fig. 93B. Total colitis in ulcerative
colitis leads to a featureless, 'hose-pipe,'
colon. Rectum involved in 95%.

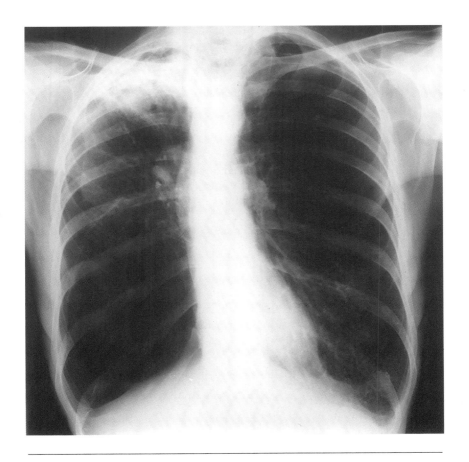

94   What is the likely cause of haemoptysis in this 50-year-old male?

94   There is a **mycetoma** (aspergilloma, fungus ball) within a pre-existing cavity in the right upper lobe (at the level of the medial end of the clavicle). Note the rounded mass of soft tissue density lying within the cavity. There is a characteristic air-crescent sign surrounding the fungus ball which does not completely fill the cavity. This sign, although not specific to mycetoma, strongly suggests the diagnosis and another useful diagnostic sign is that a fungus ball moves with patient positioning.

Pleural thickening of up to 2 cm adjacent to the cavity is a frequent finding of Aspergillus superinfection and may be the first sign in a patient with a pre-existing lung cavity. CT scanning demonstrates these features even better.

The fungus ball may calcify.

Although the pulmonary cavities are usually due to old, healed pulmonary tuberculosis (note the right upper zone fibrosis, elevation of the right hilum and hilar nodal calcification) other causes include sarcoidosis, ankylosing spondylitis and bronchiectasis. In this patient there are also large emphysematous bullae in the right lower and left upper zones, respectively.

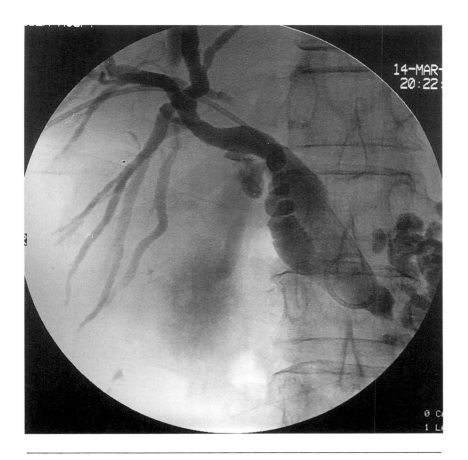

95a   What type of investigation is this?

95b   What radiological abnormality is shown?

95c   Name three causes of this appearance.

95a   A percutaneous transhepatic cholangiogram (PTC).

95b   **Obstruction of the distal common bile duct** with dilatation of the intrahepatic ducts, cystic duct, common hepatic and common bile duct. The level of obstruction is within the pancreas with abrupt tapering of the common bile duct. Multiple densities (i.e. of similar density to the dense contrast material within the bile duct), consistent with calcifications, are seen in the region of the head of pancreas, projected over the left lateral border of the lumbar vertebrae, consistent with **chronic calcific pancreatitis**. Such calcifications are seen more clearly on the preliminary plain abdominal film prior to the injection of contrast.

In this examination, a needle is passed percutaneously into the liver under local anaesthesia and contrast is injected into the biliary tree. A catheter can then be inserted to drain an obstructed system (as above).

95c   Causes of distal common bile duct obstruction include:
- Calculi: single or multiple intraluminal filling defects that may change position.
- Malignant tumours: including cholangiocarcinoma, ampullary tumours and carcinoma of the pancreas. Compression by enlarged lymph nodes.
- Chronic pancreatitis: look for pancreatic calcifications.
- Inflammatory benign strictures, e.g. due to recurrent pyogenic cholangitis, pancreatic pseudocyst, etc.

CASE 96

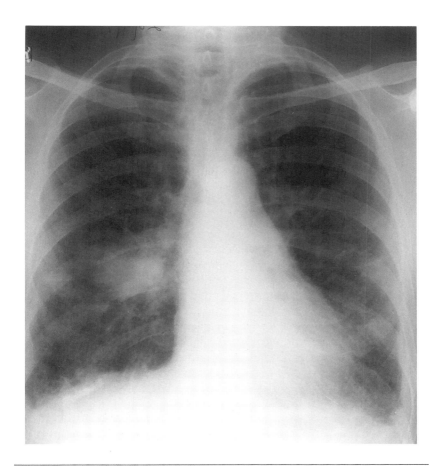

96a   What three radiological abnormalities are shown?

96b   What is the diagnosis?

96a   i) Pleural thickening and calcified pleural plaques (right hemidiaphragm).

      ii) Large, irregular, non-cavitating pulmonary mass – projected over the inferior pole of the right hilum.

      iii)A fine reticular pattern in both lower zones.

96b   **Asbestosis and a bronchogenic carcinoma.**

Plaques occur on the parietal pleura and are seen in 50% of patients exposed to asbestos (not before 20 years or more have elapsed). They tend to be multiple and favour the lower hemithorax. The interstitial, reticular pattern compatible with fibrosis (asbestosis) is typically basal. There is an increased incidence of bronchogenic carcinoma in smokers with asbestosis.

Other findings include mesothelioma (80% of all mesotheliomas are associated with asbestosis) and pleural effusions.

Pleural calcification may also be due to an old empyema, haemothorax (typically unilateral) or talc exposure (similar appearance to asbestos exposure).

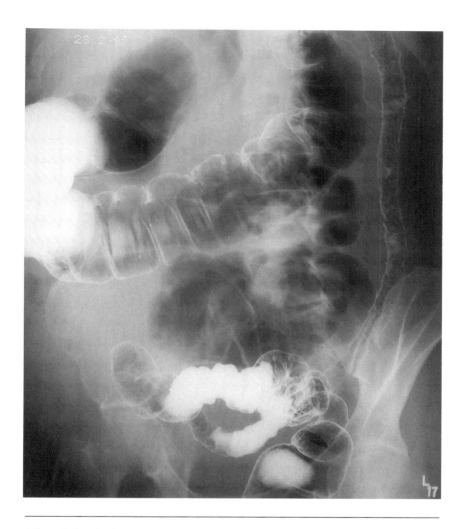

97   What is the likely cause of acute abdominal pain and rectal bleeding
      in this 72-year-old patient?

97   Ischaemic colitis

The double contrast barium enema shows a continuous long narrowed segment extending from the splenic flexure to the sigmoid colon with fine mucosal ulceration. There is no evidence of associated malignancy or diverticular disease.

The radiological findings in conjunction with the clinical history make ischaemic colitis the most likely diagnosis.

The descending colon (90%) and splenic flexure (80%) are the commonest sites of involvement in ischaemic colitis.

Plain film changes include thumb printing (marginal indentations on the mesenteric side), lack of haustration and narrowing. Barium enema is the definitive investigation (abnormal in 90% of patients) and features include superficial ulcerations, thumb printing (due to submucosal haemorrhage and oedema), and rigidity.

Poor prognostic features are those of toxic megacolon (colonic calibre greater than 5.5 cm), pneumoperitoneum and gas in the portal vein. Intramural gas may be seen and is linear in configuration rather than spherical as in pneumatosis coli (Fig. 15A).

Causes of toxic megacolon are:
- Inflammatory: ulcerative colitis, Crohn's disease and pseudomembranous colitis.
- Ischaemic colitis.
- Dysentery: amoebiasis, Salmonella.

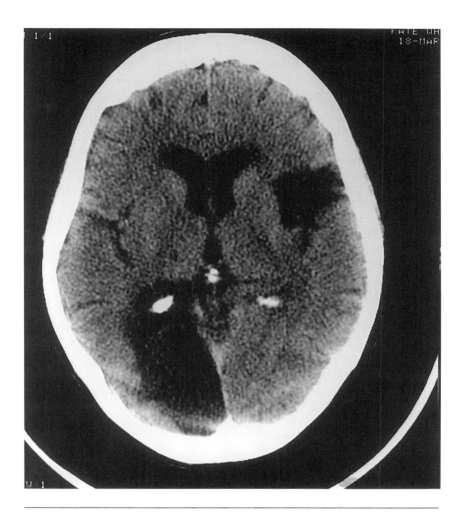

98   What is the diagnosis based on this unenhanced CT head scan of a
      70-year-old man?

98   There is a well-defined, focal area of decreased attenuation in the left frontoparietal region. There is no associated mass effect and appearances are in keeping with an **old infarct** (ischaemic lesion) in the left middle cerebral artery territory (the most common territory involved). In addition, there is asymmetrical enlargement of the posterior horn of the right lateral ventricle which is due to a previous right occipital infarct.

The CT appearances of cerebral infarction are time dependent. Unless accompanied by haemorrhage in the first 24 hours, CT will detect only 50% of infarcts. Findings include slight hypodensity, minimal mass effect and loss of distinction between grey and white matter.

Mass effect due to oedema is maximal at 3–5 days and gyriform contrast enhancement (when given) is maximal between 2–4 weeks.

Haemorrhage may occur after a few days to two weeks due to rebleeding from reperfused, damaged capillaries.

In the chronic stage (by 2–3 months post-event), a well defined low attenuation area (the same density as CSF) is seen, associated with volume loss (dilatation of adjacent ventricles and sulci).

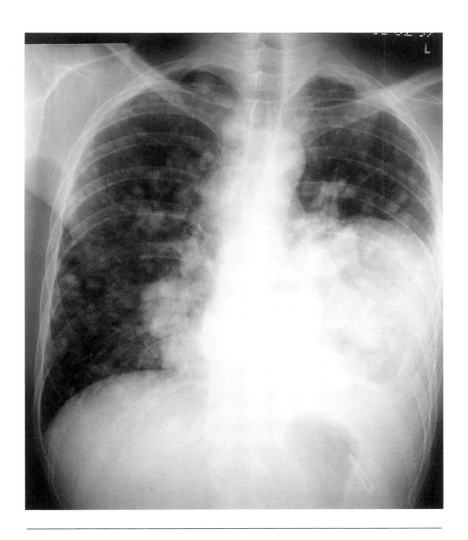

99a   Name three radiological abnormalities.

99b   What is the likely cause of these pulmonary appearances?

99a i) **Multiple pulmonary nodules** of soft tissue density and variable size (the largest is at the left base).

ii) **Small right apical pneumothorax** (absence of lung markings above the right clavicle).

iii) **Surgical blade** projected over the left hypochondrium (embedded in the left hemidiaphragm, following removal of a chest drain).

99b **Pulmonary metastases** – subpleural deposits have caused the pneumothorax.

Causes of multiple pulmonary nodules (> 5 mm) include:
- Pulmonary metastases: most commonly from breast, thyroid, gastrointestinal tract, kidney and testes. Predilection for lower lobes. Various sizes and well-defined.
- Infections: abscesses (cavitation common).
- Wegener's granulomatosis: widespread, round and well defined. No calcification. May cavitate (30–50%).
- Rheumatoid nodules: peripheral and more common in lower zones. Cavitation common.
- Caplan's syndrome: background nodularity of pneumoconiosis. Calcification and cavitation occurs.
- Progressive massive fibrosis: mid and upper zones.
- Arteriovenous malformations.

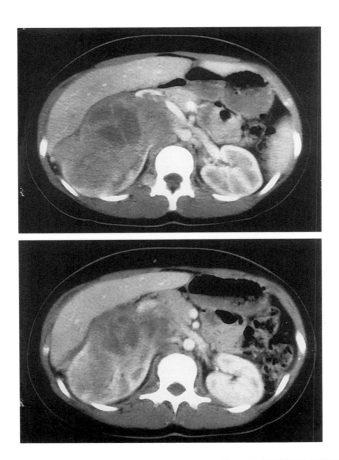

100a   What abnormality is shown on these two sections from a
       contrast-enhanced CT scan of the abdomen of a 7-year-old child?

100b   What is the most likely diagnosis?

100a   There is a large soft tissue mass of mixed attenuation arising from the right kidney. It contains low attenuation areas compatible with haemorrhage/necrosis. It extends towards the midline and displaces the right renal artery anteriorly. No calcification is seen. Although not clearly shown on these sections, the right renal vein and IVC were invaded by tumour. Normal liver and left kidney.

100b   **Wilms' tumour**

This is the commonest abdominal malignancy of childhood with 90% occurring before 8 years of age. They are bilateral in 5% of cases and typically large (average size 12 cm). Calcification is uncommon (5–10%). Five per cent have tumour thrombus in the IVC or right atrium. Ninety per cent have favourable histology.

Plain films may show a bulging flank (75%), loss of the renal outline (66%), enlargement of the renal outline, displacement of bowel gas (50%), loss of psoas outline and calcification.

On IVU (Fig. 100A) there is usually calyceal distortion, but in 10% of cases the kidney is not visualized.

Renal cell carcinoma (90% of adult malignant renal tumours) is rare in childhood and carries a worse prognosis than Wilms' tumour.

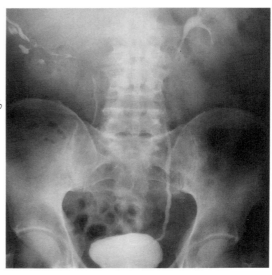

Fig. 100A. IVU. Right renal cell carcinoma (adult patient) showing calyceal distortion due to an upper pole mass.

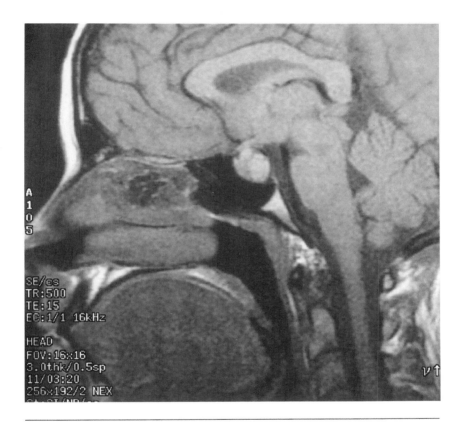

101 What abnormality is shown on this MRI scan of a 25-year-old
     female?

101 **A pituitary macroadenoma**

This T_1-weighted sagittal MRI brain scan without contrast shows enlargement of the pituitary fossa by a large pituitary mass, with suprasellar extension up to the optic chiasm.

MRI, with its multiplanar capability, is the optimal imaging technique for this region. On T_1-weighted images, pituitary tumours tend to be of slightly lower signal intensity than the adjacent anterior pituitary tissue, a difference that is emphasized after intravenous contrast enhancement, i.e. the adenoma does not enhance, but normal adjacent pituitary gland enhances substantially. The size of tumour at presentation varies from a few millimetres with adrenocorticotrophic hormone-producing adenomas to very large, in the case of non-functioning tumours or those that produce prolactin (as in this case) or growth hormone. A macroadenoma is defined as a tumour of diameter greater than 1 cm. There are no imaging features to distinguish between different types of adenoma.

Large tumours may extend upwards into the suprasellar cistern and compress the optic chiasm and hypothalamus. Invasive tumours grow into the cavernous sinus and may invade adjacent brain substance.

INDEX

The numbers in this index are the question and answer numbers.

Index

MRCP Part 2 Preparation for the Clinical Examination £14.50
Julian Gray

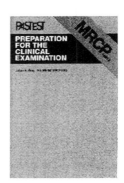

- A very popular title offering a systematic approach to preparing for the long case, short cases and viva.
- Over 120 popular Short Case topics.
- Vital hints on presentation.
- Useful schemes of clinical examination.
- Advice on methods of revision, useful lists and Revision Index.

Data Interpretation for the MCRP £15.95
Peter Clark and Roderick Neilson

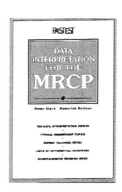

- 10 Data Interpretation practice papers with strong clinical orientation.
- Includes a wide selection of data and charts reflecting the demands of the exam.
- Correct answers and detailed teaching notes.
- Listings of Differential Diagnoses provide a useful aid to recognising specific data patterns.
- Revision Index.

MRCP Part 2 Pocket Books

£8.25 each

Series Editor R L Hawkins

- Each pocket-sized book contains Case Histories and Data Interpretations for selected subject areas.
- Questions represent favourite Membership topics.
- Correct answers and extensive teaching notes for every question.
- Revision Index for easy reference to specific topics.

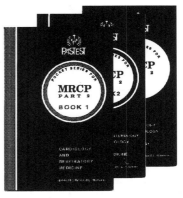

MRCP Part 2 Paediatric Practice Exams

£14.95

Deb Pal and Paul Gringas

- Five complete written papers.
- Each exam contains five Case Histories and ten Data Interpretations.
- All questions based on past Membership papers.
- Correct answers with detailed teaching notes.
- Unique Key Points sections highlight essential points for revision.
- Essential practice material for all MRCP Part 2 Paediatric candidates.

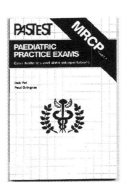

All PasTest books are available from good bookshops. For priority mail order service, telephone us at the number below or contact us by mail or fax.

PasTest, Freepost, Egerton Court, Parkgate Estate, Knutsford, Cheshire WA16 7BR, UK

Telephone: 01565 752000   Fax: 01565 650264

ORDER FORM

Please send me:
- ❏ One copy of MRCP Part 2 Preparation for the
  Clinical Examination   £14.50
- ❏ Data Interpretation for the MCRP   £15.95
- ❏ One copy of each MRCP Part 2 Pocket Books   £8.25 each
- ❏ One copy of MCRP Part 2 Paediatric Practice Exams   £14.95

Please add cost of postage:

UK: £1.50 for the first book plus £1.00 for each additional book
Europe: £2.00 for the first book plus £1.00 for each additional book
Outside Europe: £3.75 for the first book plus £2.50 for each
additional book

Name: . . . .

Address: . . . .

. . . .

. . . .

Daytime telephone: . . . .

- ❏ I enclose a cheque/money order payable in sterling to PasTest.
  Please write your cheque guarantee card number and expiry date
  clearly on the back of the cheque
- ❏ Please debit my Access/Visa/Switch card

     Card number . . . .

     Expiry date . . . . Switch Issue Number . . . .

Signature . . . .

Send this form with your payment to:

PasTest, Freepost
Knutsford, Cheshire WA16 7BR

Telephone: 01565 752000   Fax: 01565 650 264
e-mail: books@pastest.co.uk
web site: http://www.pastest.co.uk